the future. Yet performance cannot be predicted on analysis of memory, but it can actually be revealed by audit of action. The relationship between correct memory and correct action is not direct, for correct action depends partly on the proper discipline in approaching medical problems. □ 5. Also central to the educational system was the assumption that isolated facts presented by a highly specialized faculty would be synthesized and managed in an integrated fashion by practicing physicians. But synthesis itself is a sophisticated technique, and by no means may be assumed. □ 6. Far more molecular biological research was performed and the results of far more taught than could be applied meaningfully in patient care, with the result that present patients were deprived of practical medical assistance in our concern for future patients. An additional consequence was that a great deal of wisdom about the everyday care of present patients was never gained and applied. □ 7. Medical students and physicians were trained professionally without day-to-day education in the economic and cost-benefit analysis of what doctors do. As a consequence, large funds were applied to the wrong problems at the wrong times. □ 8. The characteristics of medical education and practice just described have combined to produce a non-system that now defies standardization and the sensible application of resources in a national network of information and management.

—LAWRENCE L. WEED, M.D.

MEDICAL RECORDS, MEDICAL EDUCATION, AND PATIENT CARE

LAWRENCE L. WEED, M.D.

The revolutionary system proposed in this volume can turn the patient's medical record into a dynamic instrument for structuring medical care. It raises the medical record to the level of a scientific manuscript and makes it a central tool in medical education and in quality control of medical care. The system, in addition, facilitates computerization of the medical record.

Dr. Weed's plan embodies four phases of medical action: (1) the collection of data (medical history, physical examination, and laboratory data); (2) the formulation of problems; (3) the development of plans and treatment for each problem; and, most important, (4) the follow-up through the use of numbered and titled progress notes for each problem.

Under current methods of keeping medical records, the data base for the average patient is often disorganized, incomplete, and variable in size – affected by the whims, energy level, available time, and level of training of the attending physician. Many patients, furthermore, have not one but a multitude of problems, yet their records rarely contain a complete, up-to-date list of these. Without such a list, particularly in an era of specialization, there is always the danger of neglecting some problems and therefore of treating others out of context. And finally, random, non-problem-oriented progress notes have made a meaningful audit of patient care impossible.

Medical Records, Medical Education, and Patient Care presents a plan for assembling patient data and organizing it by problem, thus ensuring a truly logical framework for the practice of medicine.

Lawrence L. Weed was formerly Medical Director, Out Patient Clinic, Cleveland Metropolitan General Hospital, and professor of medicine and associate professor of microbiology, Case Western Reserve University School of Medicine. He is now professor of medicine and professor of community medicine, and Director of the Problem-Oriented Medical Information System (PROMIS) Laboratory, College of Medicine, University of Vermont.

MEDICAL RECORDS,
MEDICAL EDUCATION,
AND PATIENT CARE

MEDICAL RECORDS, MEDICAL EDUCATION, AND PATIENT CARE

The Problem-Oriented Record as a Basic Tool

LAWRENCE L. WEED, M. D.

Professor of Medicine and Professor of
Community Medicine
Director, PROMIS Laboratory
College of Medicine
University of Vermont

The Press of Case Western Reserve University

Distributed by Year Book Medical Publishers, Inc.,
35 East Wacker Drive, Chicago

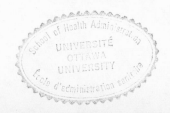

Fourth Printing

Copyright © 1969, 1970, 1971 by The Press of Case Western Reserve
University, Cleveland, Ohio 44106

Printed in the United States of America.

Standard Book Number: 8151-9188-X

Library of Congress Catalogue Card Number: 69-17686

PREFACE

If communities were the size of cells and if hospitals, pharmacies, laboratories, patients, and physicians were the size of subcellular particles, no doubt they would be the subjects of a great deal of research, and much more would be known about their interrelationships and pathophysiology. But the apparent ease with which the organization of medicine itself can be observed has discouraged examination of it and has even made the idea of that examination seem somehow naive and unscientific. Research and planning at the community level may be troublesome. Others besides you observe and are affected by what you are doing, and they are eager to point out imperfections when they see them. To deal with indirect evidence and the abstract at the molecular and microscopic level is not only sophisticated and intellectually satisfying but is a good deal safer, for imperfections are discernible to but a few, and the investigator himself sees flaws only in proportion to his capacity to develop and use analytical methods to reveal them. It is not surprising that so much of our nation's intellectual power has been directed out to space or in to the double helix, where rewards are well defined and the frustrations of dealing with a society that often seems essentially irrational and uncontrollable are largely absent. It is true that failures occur at the sophisticated levels, too, but they are made in tolerable obscurity and rarely under conditions of frustration and social unrest.

All of us would like to correct this imbalance, to see the organization of medicine well studied and well ordered, without, at the same time, shifting the weight of research and planning so far that the undeniable benefits of a concentration on specialized subject areas are lost. Indeed, not only would the standard of medical care aspired to in this volume be impossible without medicine's long history of the closely focused and theoretical study of the science of health and disease, but it is precisely in the effort to apply the fruits of that research effectively and broadly and to order and integrate the elements of it that this volume has been prepared. We cannot help solve society's everyday problems by putting people under electron microscopes or out into the Van Allen belt; we can help not only by the intelligent use of the tools of systems analysis and sociology but also by a basic realization that to improve the quality of the practice of everyday medicine is worthy of our best efforts.

Two fundamental steps in working effectively at the community level are establishing a practical system of communication for use in caring for all people and fixing the standards for such a system so that problems and progress can be defined. Central in the present system of communication is the medical record, upon which patient care, much clinical investigation, and medical education depend, and even unrefined standards lead to the conclusion that it is in need of immediate attention. In its current state it is an instrument full of serious faults, being sometimes irregular, diffuse, subjective, and incomplete. Developed standards for the preparation of the medical record do not exist. Where would biochemistry or physics be if reports of their progress depended on journals without qualified boards of editors administering developed standards? One may conjecture that progress in such fields would seriously have been retarded. There is in existence at the present time no body of literature on how to structure the medical record, particularly progress notes on long-term problems, and so there is no framework within which discipline can develop.

My thesis is that this situation can be remedied. The medical record need not be simply a static, *pro forma* repository of medical observations and activities grouped in the meaningless order of source—whether doctor or nurse, laboratory or X-ray department—rather than with respect to the problems to which they pertain; it can be problem-oriented, and thereby it can become a dynamic, structured, creative instrument for facilitating comprehensive and highly specialized medical care. But in addition to being problem-oriented, the medical record must be concise, cogent, and complete, not diffuse, superficial, or fragmentary, for the latter characteristics lead to care out of context. The medical record must serve the experienced physician and yet be intelligible to the medical student; it must serve the student and yet not frustrate the practicing physician; it must be adaptable to computerization but not require it; it must give freedom of expression to the most perceptive and experienced physician, yet must establish form and order to prevent personalization of the record to the point at which subjectivity impairs communication. The medical record must serve the patient as well as the physician, so it must be equally intelligible to all physicians, since patients are likely to require the services of many physicians and as much as possible the progress of the patient among them must be easy and without confusion. The medical record must completely and honestly convey the many variables and complexities that surround every decision, thereby discouraging unreasonable demands upon the physician for supernatural understanding and superhuman competence; but at the same time it must faithfully represent events and decisions so that errors can be detected and proper corrective measures taken when lapses in thoroughness, disciplined thought, and reasonable follow-up occur. The medical record must be the natural extension of the basic science training of the physician; in short, it must be a scientific manuscript.

The pages that follow present specific steps in record-keeping that attempt to satisfy these sometimes paradoxical requirements. They can be satisfied. The contradictions in aims are apparent, not real, as intelligent use of a well-structured, problem-oriented medical record will reveal.

*   *   *

I note that, as will readily be apparent to the reader, the records presented as examples in the text have not been revised retrospectively for the purpose of quotation here. They contain jargon and unnecessary abbreviations, and the quality of the medicine practiced and the logic displayed in the pursuit of solutions to problems are not always exemplary. Many of the problem lists are not in the exact form prescribed; and many of the progress notes, though problem-oriented, do not contain concise analytical descriptions and conclusions. However, all are real and consequently are actual, not imagined, referents to day-by-day medical practice, and all are instructive stages in the direction of the system recommended.

Most of the examples used here represent care for acute, hospital-type problems, even though the text emphasizes the need for more attention to ambulatory care and preventive medicine and demographic approaches in defining and dealing with problems. Appendix E and a forthcoming volume by two general practitioners using problem-oriented records will better illustrate this emphasis.

L.L.W.

ACKNOWLEDGMENTS

The author wishes to acknowledge the contribution of the Director, Frank Curran, and the intern staffs of the Eastern Maine General Hospital, in association with whom most of the thinking and much of the work on the problem-oriented medical record began in the years between 1956 and 1960, and the continuing contributions of Dr. Harold Cross and Dr. John Bjorn through their daily exploration of these concepts and techniques in their general practice in Hampden Highlands, Maine.

The author wishes also to acknowledge his indebtedness to the many House Officers of the Cleveland Metropolitan General Hospital who have made fundamental contributions to the concepts and contents of this book, and especially to Dr. Charles Rammelkamp, Dr. Frederick C. Robbins, and Mr. David A. Miller, each of whom did so much initially to create and support an environment in which the implications of these approaches could be freely and fully explored.

The author is grateful to Dr. T. Hale Ham, Director of the Division of Research in Medical Education, Case Western Reserve University School of Medicine, who, following his observations of the efforts at the Cleveland Metropolitan General Hospital, encouraged the preparation of this book.

The author wishes to express a particular debt of gratitude to the publisher for his expert guidance and editing, and especially for his remarkable insight into the issues and concepts with which this book is concerned.

The author is indebted to Dr. D. Wright Wilson, former chairman of the Department of Biochemistry, University of Pennsylvania School of Medicine, for his support of the author's explorations and research in the basic science aspects of medicine, and to Dr. Lester Krampitz, Chairman of the Department of Microbiology, Case Western Reserve University School of Medicine, for his generosity with time and facilities, as the author extended his efforts beyond the confines of his department and his institution.

The work on the computer applications of the medical record cited in this book was financed by a research grant from the Public Health Service, Department of Health, Education and Welfare, #5-R 18-HM-00578-02, entitled "The Automation of a Problem-Oriented Medical Record," and was done in collaboration with the Co-Principal Investigator on this project, Mr. Jan Schultz. Support was also provided in part by the National Fund for Research in Medical Education.

Publication of an earlier research-format edition was supported in part through the Division of Research in Medical Education by a grant from the Carnegie Corporation of New York and by a grant from the National Library of Medicine, Public Health Service, Department of Health, Education and Welfare, #1-RO 1-LM-00673-01, entitled "Development and Evaluation of Instructional Materials."

Finally, I am grateful to my wife for her understanding and many contributions to all these efforts.

LAWRENCE L. WEED, M.D.
Professor of Medicine and Professor of
Community Medicine
Director, PROMIS Laboratory
College of Medicine
University of Vermont

CONTENTS

LIST OF FIGURES

MEDICAL RECORDS, MEDICAL EDUCATION, AND PATIENT CARE

1

INTRODUCTION

The beginning clinical clerk, the new intern, and the practicing physician are confronted with an apparent contradiction. Each is asked, as a "whole" physician, to accept the obligations of meeting many problems simultaneously and yet to give to all the single-minded attention that is fundamental to developing and mobilizing his enthusiasm and skill—for these two virtues do not arise except where an organized concentration upon a particular subject is possible. It is this multiplicity of problems with which the physician must deal in his daily work that constitutes the principal distinguishing feature between his activities and those of many other scientists. The multiplicity is inevitable, but a random approach to the difficulties it creates is not. The instruction of physicians should be based on a system that helps them to define and follow clinical problems one by one and then systematically to relate and resolve them. Doctors vary tremendously in their capacity to deal competently with widely varying numbers and types of challenges in medical practice. We must therefore sort out physicians in terms of what they *actually do* competently for patients and not in terms of how they trained, what specialty group they joined, or how well they fared in qualifying examinations. In other words, the basic criterion of the physician is how well he can identify the patient's problems and organize them for solution.

What is done in medical education to prepare the physician for a lifelong scrutiny of the records on his patients? The answer is, very little, for in many medical schools, as in many specialty training programs, elaborate provisions are made for transmitting the facts of basic science and clinical medicine, but little is done to transmit to the student the scientific methodology that will eventually permit him to deal with complex biological systems successfully.

What is this methodology? The scientist defines a problem clearly, separates multifarious problems into their individual components, and clarifies their relationships to each other. He records data in a communicative and standard form and ultimately accepts an audit from objective peers by seeking publication in a journal. Basic scientists are neither better people nor better scholars than physicians; they do not pursue more scientific or intrinsically "better" problems. They are simply subject to better monitoring by a system that mobilizes the criticism of their peers throughout their lives. Clinical medicine, on the other hand, substitutes qualifying examinations at a single point in a career for a lifelong process of recurring audit and it must frankly be admitted that the customary methodology of medicine fails to provide the kind of structured context that promotes objectivity, sharpens skills, and permits progressive self-evaluation.

To focus the comparison more sharply, let us look at the clinical specialty board candidate and the basic science graduate-degree aspirant. The latter, after spending the first year or two mainly in course work, devotes an increasing proportion of his time to his thesis, to which all his other activities ultimately become secondary. Conferences, seminars, normal free time—all are set aside, if need be, because it is by his thesis that the candidate scientist will be judged. The thesis reveals both what he knows and what he is capable of doing with what he knows. Each day, as he works, his preceptor and his colleagues can study and criticize his data as he records them in his notebooks. Finally, everyone who sits on his examination board reviews a copy of his thesis, which is written in a very standard form so as to simplify critical analysis, as a precondition of acceptance. If he receives his degree, he proceeds to a new problem, completes his research on it, prepares his report, and submits it for publication to a journal whose editors exercise the right to establish standards of form and content and may require him to rewrite his paper several times. As a consequence of this process, he develops a respect for order, logic, and consistency and cooperates with his critics without feeling that his creativity and originality are jeopardized by their guidance. It would not occur to the scientist to protest to the editors that there is much "art" in his laboratory work that never can be recorded and that the editors have to see him at work in order fully to appreciate him.

The clinical specialty board candidate, on the other hand, submits to examinations in which he is asked to recall memorized facts. No thesis composed of analyses and defenses of his cases recorded in a specific form is required of him. Instead, he is given an informal oral examination on the basis of a preselected case; preselected data are presented to him in a setting bearing little relationship to the realities of the clinical setting in which patients are normally "worked up" in the clinic and in the ward. The strategy and completeness of his own search for the data, the depth of his theoretical understanding and the delicacy of the analytical capacity that will permit him to make sound therapeutic decisions, and his ability to sustain quality and energy in his daily attack on all types of problems, esoteric and mundane, are poorly evaluated by such examining procedures.

In clinical situations there is in effect not a single thesis, but there are a thousand of them. Little time can be devoted to each, and the physician is confronted with biological variables that are exceptionally difficult to enumerate and control and that are complicated by concurrent human and social problems. The need for organization grows with increasing complexity and pressure of time. Yet the intellectual discipline addressed to clinical problems is often superficial; documentation may be haphazard; systems are ill-defined; and no audit ever takes place.

Figure 1 is a partial sequence of notes extracted from a complicated, unstructured record of a patient with a long list of problems. Facts are presented in language that suggests difficulties in many systems, but the record is so confused, is such a tangle of illogically assembled bits of information, that one cannot reliably discern from it how (or whether) the physician defined and logically pursued each problem.

A double standard exists. We invoke discipline when we prepare the manuscript concerning laboratory research, and we abandon discipline when we write final progress notes, such as these, on the care of patients. The care itself may suffer. The confidence of those students who observe our failure to discipline ourselves also suffers.

We can help students systematize their clinical experience by means of their clinical records; we can demand that they present the data they accumulate on each problem in a consistent, well-organized form, clearly delineated. That this can be done is shown by an extension of the record in Fig. 1; this extension, presented as Fig. 2, was prepared by a second physician, who assumed responsibility for the same case. Under the new physician, the situation abruptly changed, and the titles of each of the progress notes at once began to make clear the total nature of the case. For example, if we focus on a single problem (#2b. RLL pneumonia), we are immediately able to assess the quality of patient care. We know what attention is or is not being paid to the patient's symptoms, physical findings, and sputum characteristics. We can observe what steps have or have not been taken for the physical management of the patient and in particular what has been done, if anything, to assure the proper drainage of his chest.

If we fail to provide a system for—and to demand order from—students and physicians, then we should not be surprised if they reveal anxiety and confusion in the management of complicated cases. The recourse for many of them is to seek shelter in specialization, where single-mindedness is acceptable and multifarious problems may be ignored.

The education of a physician for specialized and for total care should be based on his own clinical experience and should be reflected in the records he maintains on his patients. An educational institution should set the pattern for the physician's professional development, and the pattern should be based not on grand rounds,

9/10

Patient received 40 units of regular insulin yest. because of B & 4+ urine sugars. Got 2000 cc Amigen yest. & 500 cc D5W. Was febrile all night up to 40 at 8PM; this gradually came down to 39. 8PM yest. suctioned & coughed up $\bar{c}$ return of $\frac{1}{2}$ cup of thick white sputum—cultured also blood cultures. Was in must. tent $\bar{c}$ mucomist overnight. At 4PM yest. had B-R base. Sputum smear unremarkable—WBC's but no bacteria.

9/10—12:30

10 o'clock urine 2-3+/0. Given 10 U. reg. ins. at 12:30 PM. Temp. down to 38? Suctioned N.T. $\bar{c}$ little return. However during suctioning pt. vomited 100-150 cc green fluid. Proximal jejunostomy tube draining well now.

9/11—9 AM

Urine 3+ given 10 U reg. insulin. Pt. was hiccuping all night & this AM. Levine tube passed $\bar{c}$ 900-1000 cc bileous fluid removed. Jejunostomy tubes have been draining minimally. Will have Levine tube down.

   /Three pages of similar notes follow until 9/26/

9/26

Last night 10PM had seizure like behavior and acting strange. Apparently hallucinating. Blood sugar didn't register on destrostix. Had been given 10 units reg. insulin at 8 PM after IV glucose returned to nl¶ This AM vomited up brown black fluid 300 cc + for occult blood. NG tube had been out since 5PM yest. NG tube replaced & some material small amt. withdrawn. Pt. now NPO $\bar{c}$ NG tube to Gomco.

9/27

Still febrile—Ampicillin 1g qid—continued; Blood cult. drawn to check if septicemia still present. Chest X ray today shows infiltrate in (R) lower lobe. No effusion. Sputum grew out pseudomonas but Dr. —— elected not to treat this.

FIGURE 1. Unstructured patient record. The facts presented suggest difficulties in many systems but the information is so illogically grouped that one cannot reliably discern if the physician defined each problem correctly or pursued each problem logically. The record is reproduced as originally phrased, without editing ($\bar{c}$ = with).

10/2—6PM

#1 Chronic Relapsing Panc.:

b. Diabetes: will continue moment to moment Rx of spot urines for
    now. Today $\bar{c}$ only 10 regular insulin pt. spilling mainly 2-3+.
    Plan: BLD sugar tomorrow

c. Panc. insuff.: will begin Cotazyn-B

#2 Complications Following Laparotomy:

c. Post op ileus: KUB tomorrow. Pt. now tolerating ice cream and
    occ. candy. bs. poor; $\bar{s}$ gross distention; stool passes regu-
    larly ⟶ fistula
    Imp: prob. resolving now
    Plan: KUB and continue small feedings

d. Sepsis: afebrile now on Ampicillin. see flow sheet. Reculture
    tomorrow.

b. RLL Pneumonia: Film of 9/28 shows some ↑ in this process. Will
    repeat P.A. chest tomorrow & cultures.

e. Colonic-Cutaneous Fistula: Continues to drain semi-formed stool
    several times per day; the problem is that stool drains onto
    granulating abd. wound.
    Plan: culture stool; Remove some non-func stay sutures; Freq
    dressings & consider colostomy bag for fistula.

10/3

#1 Chronic Relapsing Panc.:

c. Panc. insufficiency: Cotazyn-B will be begun (special purchase)
    and will evaluate effect on absorption and/or stool content by
    measuring amt. of fat.

FIGURE 2. Problem-oriented patient record, a continuation of Fig. 1,
prepared by a second physician after reading the following instruction,
which was written into the record: "Please read revised problem list and
please use #'s shown." Numbers refer to a numbered problem list of the
type described in Chapter 3. The record is reproduced without editing
($\bar{c}$ = with; $\bar{o}$ = none, no; $\bar{s}$ = without).

f. Pain: pt. still requires freq narcotics. Neurosurg will eventually perform epidural block and depending upon results will consider cordotomy.

#2 Complications Following Laparotomy:

b. RLL Pneumonia: Chest X-ray today shows marked resolution of previously described infiltrates; pt. has been afebrile—sputum recultured (see #2).

c. Post op ileus: KUB today shows little improvement from film of 9/29. Ba in same position in colon which is distal to fistula. Despite this X-ray findings will continue to feed (see #2f). Bowel sounds poor and abd. seems slightly more distended. Will give oil retention enema to try to clear distal colon.

d. Sepsis: Pt. has been afebrile, cultures repeated today; ō (M) heard today; has been on Ampicillin x 9 days. Although potential still present this problem is under relatively good control.

e. Colonic-Cutaneous Fistula: all stay sutures removed today and wound is well granulated but constantly bathed c̄ stool. Colostomy bag applied to try to control this drainage. Etiology of fistula? but may be serving decompressive function.

f. Malnutrition: Total protein = 6.1 c 2.1/4.0 = A/G in 1965. Wt. has ↓ from 141# ⟶ 113# since adm.

Imp: little resolution of ileus, in fact, most of food stays in stomach probably; this remains the main problem; other as above fairly well controlled except malnutrition.

Plan: as above plus give gastro-graffin per NG tube and watch progress; avoid surgery.

FIGURE 2 (Continued)

conferences, and journal clubs but on a detailed scrutiny of the clinical experience of students, house officers, and staff, as the clinical records reveal it. The education of a student, a resident physician, or a senior physician becomes defective not when he is given too much or too little training in basic science nor when his clinical load falls below an ideal standard but rather when he is allowed to ignore or slight the elementary definition and the progressive adjustment of the problems that comprise his clinical experience. The teacher* who ultimately benefits students most is the one who is willing to establish parameters of discipline in the not unsophisticated but often unappreciated task of preventing this imprecision and disorganization. Avoiding irrelevant displays of fact, he must continually emphasize the enumeration, evaluation, integration, and continuing audit of all the patient's problems.

Problem-oriented medical records can become a vehicle for converting a broad philosophy of education into specific, attainable goals. Through the creation of a proper record and the proper management of that record, the physician's actual performance in given areas can be exposed to critical evaluation in the same way that the scientist's work is evaluated by journal editors; the physician can be assisted to demonstrate thoroughness and reliability in the formulation of all of the patient's problems; and he can be guided in the exercise of sound analytical thought, coupled with good clinical judgment, in establishing patient-care plans and in following up patient progress in each problem area.

Special cases encountered within the daily routine will always provide an unsurpassed opportunity to instruct and evaluate the physician. The same combination of variables rarely repeats itself in textbook fashion in any one case, and the manner in which the student or physician finds his way among each new combination of variables within the constant framework of sound physiological principles and avoids premature diagnostic and therapeutic decisions is the best measure of his performance and growth. Progress notes and operative notes are replete with teaching opportunities,

* "Teacher," as used in this book, includes everyone from the intern who helps the student to the full professor who teaches at many levels.

because they are relevant to the current intellectual and emotional concerns of the student or house officer who wrote them. No matter how elegant the teacher's presentation, its effect may be severely reduced if it has no connection with the student's problems at the time. The teacher will be more likely to achieve solid educational goals if he approaches the student through the specific realities that confront him at that point, using terms consistent with the student's level of understanding.

The techniques for putting this approach into effect are not difficult, so long as the teacher agrees to present facts and principles as adjuncts of concrete experience, entering the student's mind at the level it understands. If the teacher does otherwise, he may erect a superstructure of abstract information in the student's mind that is confirmed by tradition, that passes for education, but that, when the student is confronted with a particular set of variables and needs to take meaningful action, may crumble and leave him anxious and confused. Furthermore, teaching that is not based upon real physical and biological problems requiring specific solution denies not only the student but also the teacher the progressive opportunity to correct the unsound theories, the false generalizations, and the outright errors that abound in every field of knowledge. The solution of real problems is, I believe, the foundation of student morale, and by no means impedes development at the theoretical level but perhaps even enhances it.

Until our basic commitment is to the teaching of discipline and a rigorous approach to medical problems, instead of non-problem-oriented feats of memory, not only will we be unable to take advantage of the enlarged capabilities of the new generation of premedical students and reduce what is now an intolerably long training period but also we may sink deeper into the quagmire of raw information upon which our footing is already insecure, for the number of facts the memory-oriented faculty can impose upon the minds of students is limitless. The problem-oriented record, combined with almost any patient with complex problems, is uniquely suited as a vehicle for teaching approaches and essential skills, leaving libraries and computers to supply raw information and rapid retrieval. In this approach, the training period can simply be defined as that time necessary for a student to demonstrate, through a series of patient records, competence in dealing with new medical situations, using the literature and laboratories as needed.

If the role the medical record will play in his education is carefully stated to the student, the goals become clear to him as well as his teacher, and precise goals are fundamental in effective education. There must be one standard of quality for all kinds of patients: for the patient in the emergency room, the ward, or the recovery room; for the general surgical and medical clinic patient, as well as for the patient in the specialty clinic; and for all of the problems of any given patient, the mundane disorder, the esoteric diagnostic problem, the minor illness, or the major illness. The total job that needs to be done, and not merely the areas of the individual physician's or student's special interest, should be confronted head-on.

I recognize that no mere system of recording data will dispel the tragedy and confusion that surround the desperately ill. As Dr. Dickinson Richards has said, "So often the patient and doctor are waging an unequal struggle against a bitter and irrevocable fate."* Uncontrollable forces are omnipresent in the lives of all of us, excessively so in the lives of some. No system can in itself alter this human condition, but if we do our best to define all the patient's problems and to follow them up one by one, we can, with a clear conscience, set aside medical chores for a moment and be physicians in the broadest sense—and that presumably is what brought many of us into our profession in the first place. There is nothing more tragic than the "brilliant" specialist, overconfident of his knowledge and techniques, who, failing to comprehend the nature of his responsibility, fails also to treat the trusting patient in the light of his total needs.

In the practice of medicine, both intellectually and "artistically," the greatest constraint on the realization of our potential as physicians is not system, which makes data meaningful and immediately comprehensible, but disorder, which obscures forever original pat-

* D. W. Richards, "Homeostasis: Its Dislocations and Perturbations," *Perspectives in Biology and Medicine*, 3:238, 1960.

terns of thought and insight. Demand for explicit expression does not impair the quality of our perceptions; it sharpens and preserves that quality for others to build on.

THE PATIENT'S RECORD

If we are to organize the patient's record logically and efficiently, four basic elements of that record must be recognized:

1. *The Data Base.* Ordinarily present in the admission note, this may include any or all of the following: chief complaint, patient profile and related social data, present illness, past history and systems review, physical examination, and reports of laboratory work.

2. *The Problem List.* On the patient's admission to the hospital, a numbered list of problems is drawn up, containing every problem in the patient's history, past and present. New problems should be added as identified.

3. *The Initial Plan.* The next step is the preparation of a list of plans—diagnostic and therapeutic orders—for each problem, keyed by number to the original problem list.

4. *Progress Notes.*

a. *Narrative Notes.* Each progress note is related directly to the list of problems and should be numbered and titled accordingly. Operative notes and notes by nurses and paramedical personnel are to be included.

b. *Flow Sheets.* "Flow sheets" containing all the moving parameters should be kept on all problems where data and time relationships are complex. The flow sheets and the progress notes constitute the follow-up phase of the record-keeping process and, as such, are the dynamic center of the medical record.

c. *Discharge Summary.* No patient should be discharged until the house officer of the hospital has written an adequate retrospective note on each numbered problem on the patient's list.

These elements may schematically be represented as follows:

I. *Establishment of a Data Base*
History
Physical Examination
Admission Laboratory
Work

II. *Formulation of All Problems*
Problem List

III. *Plans for Each Problem*
Collection of Further
Data
Treatment
Education of Patient

IV. *Follow-up on Each Problem*
Progress Notes: Titled
and Numbered

2

THE DATA BASE

There is now little standardization among physicians in the establishment of a data base. As a consequence, correct formulation and management of all of the patient's problems are not assured. Though an imprecisely defined "routine" completeness is expected in the patient's history and physical examination regardless of specific indications, initial laboratory determinations are in fact sporadically and arbitrarily performed "only when indicated." Subclinical disease may thereby be missed, even though excessive and inappropriately selected follow-up laboratory and X ray examinations for the problems clinically evident are ordered. Thoroughness and design in the whole process decrease drastically as patient load and specialization increase, so that finally there may be observed among practicing physicians a remarkable spectrum of behavior in establishing a patient's data base—from the compulsively elaborate to the chronically haphazard. Failure to define the initial data base is like playing football with a different number of men each time on a field of no definite length. Individual plays can be perfected, but their value is unclear because their context is not constant and complete. That is, an incomplete medical exploration of the patient, which moreover may be incomplete in infinitely variable ways from patient to patient, damages the physician's ability both

15

to determine what it is he ought to do and then to assess the quality of what he actually has done.

For our purposes we shall define the data base as: (1) chief complaint; (2) patient profile (a description of how he spends his average day) and related social data; (3) present illness or illnesses; (4) past history and systems review based on a series of explicit and related questions logically arranged in a branching pattern; (5) physical examination of defined content; and (6) base-line laboratory examination.

In the light of the difficulties and dangers an uncertain definition of the size and quality of the data base may create, I take it as a principle that the initial collection of data should be as complete as possible. The only limitations should be discomfort, hazard, and expense to the patient. Advances in interview techniques and computer technology have given promise that comprehensive historical data can be acquired and stored cheaply and accurately without making insupportable inroads upon physician time. That such is already the case is strongly suggested by the work of Collen *et al.*, Slack *et al.*, and Mayne and Wedsel*—and by the results of the present utilization, at Cleveland Metropolitan General Hospital, of trained paramedical personnel as interviewers and of electronic data processing as the basic tool in recording and printing narrative data on the patient's history.

Paramedical personnel, employing meticulously refined questionnaires, assisted by automatic machines for inputting, relating, and recording information, using electronic instruments for studying all systems (particularly the cardiovascular system) and simple routines to assess the musculoskeletal system, can create a sound data base rapidly and acurately.

Nurses, properly trained, can perform entirely satisfactory breast, abdominal, and pelvic examinations. They already do Papanico-

* M. F. Collen, L. Rubin, and L. Davis, "Computers in Multiphasic Screening," in *Computers in Biomedical Research*, New York, Academic Press, 1965, Chapter 14; W. B. Slack, G. P. Hicks, C. E. Reed, and L. J. Van Cura, "Computer-Based Medical-History System," *New England Journal of Medicine*, 274:194, 1966; J. G. Mayne and W. Wedsel, "Automating the Medical History," *Mayo Clinic Proceedings*, 43 (1):1, 1968.

laou smears for interpretation by nonmedical cytologists. Sufficiently well instructed, they and other paramedical personnel can be assigned a greatly expanded role in the data-collection phase.

Once the desirable data base has been defined, individual modifications in it should not be allowed, even as rationalizations proceeding from limitations on staff time or other troublesome professional circumstances. Uniformity in data base is among the important factors tending to permit accurate comparability and generalization, and it is essential to the welfare of the whole patient. Both for the sake of our science and the sake of our patients, the standard data base must conscientiously be sought on each patient, even if paramedical personnel must ultimately be relied on to procure it. Failure to utilize paramedical personnel in the past is not, I believe, related to any intrinsic inability on their part; rather it stems from our failure to define specific goals for them and to perfect the techniques that should be applied to reach those goals. What the elements of the data base are that should be obtained by paramedical personnel is a matter that ought to remain circumstantial, but a standardized physical examination should be performed on every patient, without significant portions being omitted at the whim of the examiner. Laboratory and X-ray procedures should likewise be defined for the ideal initial data base and then carried out consistently in specific cases as they arise.

The laboratory aspects of the data base are currently under study by many scholars. Each institution and individual practitioner can contribute to this effort by keeping significant data on large series of patients on whom particular laboratory procedures have been performed, so that their comparative value can be determined. At present a complete blood count, serology, urinalysis, chest X ray, and electrocardiograph for all patients over forty, are accepted by most hospitals as routine parts of the initial data base. Vital capacity and peak flow measurement, tonometry, and Papanicolaou smears can easily be added (and should be) by almost all practitioners. Blood glucose, cholesterol, uric acid, calcium, blood urea nitrogen or creatinine, total protein with albumin/globulin ratio and electrolytes should all be routine, especially if automated facilities are available. The possible gains easily outweigh the minimal expense.

Two portions of the data base, patient profile and statement of present illness, require more detailed discussion.

Patient Profile

Much is being written today about the importance in the formulation of realistic therapeutic goals of the physician's understanding of the "whole patient" in his life situation. Yet it is extraordinary how very few clinical histories contain anything but the most desultory, insensitive "social history" sections (of the "2 packs a day, moderate drinking, born in Alabama" type), obscurely located in the patient's record. An easy remedy is the insertion, at the beginning of the history, of an explicit account of how the patient spends his routine day. Only this type of information permits the physician to plan realistically and sympathetically for the practical welfare of the patient. The two examples cited in Fig. 3 illustrate the kind of patient profile, written routinely on actual cases, that will present some significant guidance to the physician.

Statement of Present Illness

The statement of present illness should be the record of the relevant facts about a problem or a series of problems. Each problem should be discussed separately. All available information concerning a given problem should be presented, whether it comes from the patient, a relative, a friend, an old chart, a laboratory data book, a pathology slide cabinet, or the files in an X ray department. If particular information is believed to be of doubtful reliability, either that doubt becomes an important element of the related statement or the statement is altogether omitted.

Present illnesses fall roughly into two categories: those in which the problem is undiagnosed and begins with a complaint or an abnormal finding, and those that result from relapses in already well-established chronic disorders, such as rheumatic heart disease or myocardial infarction with heart failure, diabetes, and peripheral

Profile A
5/22

Intern's Readmission Note:

69-year-old married white male with known lymphocytic lymphoma was discharged 4/11, rehospitalized with comment: "I don't want to croak at home."

Information:

Patient, and wife (reliable), old chart, Dr. —— to be contacted.

Patient Profile:

Mr. —— is a 69-year-old married white male, the father of three children (with two daughters living, the son having been killed in World War II), who worked in "structural steel" and as a truck driver. He is described by his wife as a moody, somewhat self-centered individual whose main interest in life involved keeping his car (Chevy) clean and polished and going for drives in it—which he has been unable to do during the last few weeks of his illness. Recently he has been lying in bed at home, doing essentially nothing—does not read, watch TV, etc.—becoming more and more depressed, complaining of feeling weak. He is a meticulously clean person who was disturbed by the lack of cleanliness at the hospital during his previous admission, and is the type of person who is overconcerned at the slightest sign of physical illness (scratch on skin). Although he has been said to have been told his diagnosis (according to wife), he gave no evidence of knowing it during our interview (denial?).

FIGURE 3. Patient profiles.

Profile B
7/22

<u>SMS Admission Note</u>

This is the first ——— Hospital admission for this 35-year-old white
female admitted through the Gastrointestinal Clinic for therapy for a
gastric ulcer. <u>The patient's chief complaint is "my ulcer."</u>

<u>Source of Information</u>: Patient (reliable), and Outpatient Clinic
chart.

<u>Patient Profile</u>:

Mrs. ——— was born in Wilmington, Delaware—eldest of 2 children. She
attended school through 2 years of high school. She has been married
for 12 years and has no children. She and her husband lived in Wilmington until 3 years ago when they moved to Detroit so that her husband
could find a better job. They left Detroit 1 month ago because they
"hated it" and moved to Cleveland. Mr. ——— is currently employed at
C——————— and S———Company as a supervisor. He works a night shift
and is rarely at home. His income is sufficient to support them and
they have hospitalization insurance. The couple lives in a 4-room
rented apartment on West 25th St. Mrs. ——— describes herself as "a
nervous person" who worries about "little things." She has been employed for 2 weeks at L——K————Mills and says she enjoys the
work because "she can talk to the girls." Previous to this she spent
most of her time at home reading, watching TV. She notes that it is
very lonely with her husband at work most of the time and states that
she doesn't know any of her neighbors because she "doesn't mix well
with people." Up until 5 weeks ago she had a dog who was her constant
companion and whom she loved "like a little child." Her dog "passed
away" and she dissolves into tears each time she speaks about her pet.
She is quite anxious about her hospital stay—she is worried that her
ulcer will not heal, that she will need an operation, and that she
won't be able to relax properly. She knows every detail about her
illness and is extremely talkative. She does not drink alcohol but
smokes 1+ packs of Camels per day for many years. Notes that unless
she has her cigarettes at her bedside she gets extremely nervous.

FIGURE 3 (Continued)

Intern's Admission Note:

67-yr.-old white male admitted from OPC for elective T.E.A. of (R) superf. femoral artery.

#2 Generalized arteriosclerosis c̄ localized block at superf. femoral on (R):

Subj. About 5 years ago had episode of gangrene (R) 5th toe and was admitted to —— Hospital where p̄ conservative Rx apparently failed and Dr. —— performed (R) lumbar sympathectomy which also failed to heal toe. Subsequently lost (R) 5th toe surgically but still didn't heal well and was admitted to —— under Dr. ——'s care where ulcer healed with consérvative Rx. Since then has noted slow healing on feet; had (R) common fem. arteriogram 5 yrs. ago under Dr. ——'s direction; p̄ translumbar arteriogram failed (these records of five years ago are lost currently and pt. gives this info.).

FIGURE 4. Statement of present illness of a patient by a busy intern in a large urban hospital. For discussion, see text. The statement has been reproduced without editing. Abbreviations as follows:

BM = bowel movement	p = after
BP = blood pressure	P = popliteal
BUN = blood urea nitrogen	P.E. = physical examination
c̄ = with	pt = patient
DP = dorsalis pedis	PT = post tibial
ETOH = alcohol (ethanol)	qd = each day
F = femoral	(R) = right
FBS = fasting blood sugar	Rx = treatment
fem = femoral	S/P = status post
hct = hematocrit	superf = superficial
h/o = history of	T.E.A. = thromboendarectomy
IVP = intravenous pyelogram	U/A = urinalysis
(L) = left	UGI = upper gastrointestinal series
LFT = liver function test	
neg = negative	UTI = urinary tract infection
ō = none, no	WNL = within normal limits
ōr = nor	

About one year ago noted onset of severe claudication (R) leg $\bar{p}$ $\frac{1}{2}$
block and a little later "burning pain" on sole of foot. To the
present this has worsened slightly. Since that time followed con-
servatively in OPC. Smokes 1-2 packs/day; denies ETOH'ism.

<u>Obj</u>. 11/28/66 had (R) common fem. arteriogram showing local block
between middle and distal 1/3 of superf. femoral.

Pulses in OPC -		F	P	DP	PT
11/18/67	(R)	2+	-	-	-
	(L)	1+	-	-	-
10/26/66	(R)	2+	-	?+	?+
	(L)	2+	-	?+	?+

Never any ulcers noted on feet in last 1 yr. of OPC visits

<u>Rx</u>. pain meds, foot hygiene

<u>Negs</u>. neg Kline test (1966); $\bar{o}$ h/o diabetes

FBS = 98 in 1966; $\bar{o}$ pain $\bar{c}$ elevation

denies trauma

<u>#1 S/P CVA 17 yrs. ago</u>:

Residual (L) hemiparesis and tremor (L) leg - takes Dilantin for this.
$\bar{o}$ double vision, headaches, or dizziness. $\bar{o}$ loss of consciousness.

<u>#3 Labile hypertension</u>:

<u>Subj</u>. none

<u>Obj</u>. $\bar{o}$ cardiomegaly 1 yr. ago by X ray

EKG—sinus tachycardia early 1966
—WNL late 1966

BUN—15 in 1966; Cr = 1.0, 1966

U/A in 1966 = WNL

BP last admission ranged = 190-140/70-110

Last BP recorded 10/66 = 140/80

<u>Rx</u>. none

<u>#4 Benign Prostatic Hypertrophy</u>:

<u>Subj</u>. frequency, urgency, and ↓ stream x 1-2 years. nocturia x 3;
$\bar{o}$ dysuria

FIGURE 4 (Continued)

Obj. residual in 1966 = 120 cc, IVP 1966 - WNL. cystoscopy in 1966 =
median lobe impingement on urethra.

S/P open biopsy in 1966 because of nodule (R) felt by rectal ——
benign prost. hypertrophy. acid phosphotase = WNL x 2; bone series -
negative

Rx. none right now

Negs. ō h/o UTI's in recent or remote past

#5 (L) inguinal hernia—reducible:

Subj. ō

Obj. noted on P.E. in 1966

Rx. none

Negs. ō vomiting, pain, or trouble c̄ BM's

#6 H/O peptic ulcer disease:

Subj. has had pain in past in epigastrium and in p̄ 1 month it has been
worse; burning awakens him at night. relieved in AM by food; coffee
and cigarettes make ō difference. position makes ō difference; says
he's had dark black-brown stool x 1 month. Says he had UGI 5 years
ago which showed "very small" ulcer "which Dr. —— said not to worry
about."

Obj. Hct 1966 early = 46-36%

Hct 1966 late = 45%

ō guaiacs available; LFT's 1966 = WNL

Rx. Maalox——▶relief

Negs. ō food intolerance, vomiting, diarrhea, jaundice, chills, or
fever

FIGURE 4 (Continued)

vascular disease. In the first category, the statement should begin with a title, perhaps derived from the chief complaint (such as "abdominal pain"), and the history should then be recorded chronologically. Figure 4 is the statement of present illness of a patient being seen by a busy intern on the surgical service of a large urban hospital. It can be seen that this intern portrays the present illness in terms of specific problems, discussing the major problem for this particular admission first, even though that problem is the second one on the original problem list. In the second category of present illnesses, the paragraph should be titled with the disease process itself. In both categories the statement consists of: (1) symptomatic information, e.g., details concerning pain; (2) objective data, e.g., a gastrointestinal series from an old record or another hospital; (3) information concerning previous treatment, e.g., patient on Maalox; and (4) a statement of significant negatives, e.g., no blood in stools or no dark urine. In the past it has been customary to interweave information of these four types on a principle of exact chronology. There are many advantages to recording these four types separately, however: omissions are much more readily apparent, and the relative balance of symptomatic data versus objective data is quickly discerned. Also, the analytical capacity and the command of information of the student or physician are revealed as he selects and groups his facts and chooses the significant negatives. It is not true that physicians take or review histories without making choices. No one ever records all that a patient says or does, nor does anyone carry forward all the facts from previous records. Analysis and selection are always present, and the degree to which analysis and selection are done with intelligence, discrimination, and thoroughness is explicitly revealed in a structured account of the present illness.

3

THE PROBLEM LIST

The first page of the patient record should consist of a numbered problem list. It is a "table of contents" and an "index" combined, and the care with which it is constructed determines the quality of the whole record. Inherent in the problem-oriented approach to data organization in the medical record is the necessity for completeness in the formulation of the problem list and careful analysis and follow-through on each problem, as revealed in the titled progress notes. The precision of titled, problem-oriented progress notes and conclusions is directly related to the precision and integrity with which the problems are initially defined.

The student or physician should list *all* the patient's problems, past as well as present, social and psychiatric as well as medical. The list should not contain diagnostic guesses; it should simply state the problems at a level of refinement consistent with the physician's understanding, running the gamut from the precise diagnosis to the isolated, unexplained finding. The teacher should demand that the student understand a problem and be honest as he defines it, no matter how elementary the terms required. Only when both student and teacher are absolutely honest in clearly defining their level of understanding can they become intellectual colleagues, sharing thought and action in the solution of problems.

The physician or student should first ask himself as he proceeds to define a problem: Is it a medical or a social problem? If it is medical, he should classify it as *one* of the following: (1) a diagnosis, e.g., arteriosclerotic heart disease (ASHD), followed by the principal manifestation that requires management, e.g., heart failure; (2) a physiological finding, e.g., heart failure, followed by either the phrase "etiology unknown" or "2° to a diagnosis," e.g., ASHD; (3) a symptom or a physical finding, e.g., shortness of breath; or (4) an abnormal laboratory finding, e.g., an abnormal EKG.

If a given diagnosis has several major manifestations, each of which requires individual management and separate, carefully delineated progress notes, e.g., ASHD with heart failure and a supraventricular tachycardia, then the second manifestation is presented as a second problem and designated as secondary to the major diagnosis, as follows:

Problem #1. ASHD with heart failure.

Problem #2. Supraventricular tachycardia—2° to Problem #1.

If the physician thinks in terms of the requirements of proper management and his later need for logical progress notes, there need be little difficulty in determining a satisfactory problem list. Indeed, such a system immediately identifies those difficulties that have assumed major management proportions. For example, the list for one patient with cirrhosis may consist of a single problem:

Problem #1. Cirrhosis manifest by jaundice and ascites (minimal) in which management involves treatment consistent with early-stage disease.

In another patient with cirrhosis, the list may be better stated as:

Problem #1. Cirrhosis manifest by jaundice.

Problem #2. Ascites—2° to Problem #1.

In the latter case the ascites is a major problem that requires very careful diet regulation, paracentesis or diuretics, significant periods of hospitalization, even consultation for surgery. By these simple techniques the magnitude of a problem is easily discerned, and we avoid the confusion that results when we are dealing with diagnostic entities that have different manifestations, which may or may not become major management situations in themselves.

If the problem is a social one, it should be defined no less honestly and precisely, e.g., illegitimate pregnancy, bankruptcy, or severe delinquency in school. Precision in the progress notes follows from the precision with which the problems are initially defined.

As the problem is clarified, altered, or diagnosed, the original list should be modified accordingly. This modification is accomplished not by erasure but simply by the insertion of an arrow (as in Figs. 2 and 4), followed by the new diagnosis or by "dropped" or "resolved." Each change should be dated. In this manner, a record of the student's or physician's thought process is preserved. When several problems turn out to be separate manifestations of a single problem, such as a "pericarditis" and an "arthritis" becoming "lupus," then the two may be grouped together and designated as "lupus," using the number and position of the first of the two problems. The unused number then becomes inactive for all subsequent admissions and clinic visits. One may choose to keep findings separate for purposes of good management and for satisfactory progress notes, as already recommended, but, in the case above, for instance, it should be clearly stated on the original problem list that each finding is secondary to "lupus." When a new problem appears it should be added to the list and dated accordingly.

Twenty-four hours should be allowed to reformulate the initial problem list where necessary. This interval enables attending physicians, chief residents, and consultants to provide maximal help in devising the best possible definitions of all the problems. (It may be remarked that procuring definitions of this kind should be a major goal of clinical teaching.) Deciding what is wrong with the patient and in what direction medical energies should be expended is of great value both to the patient and the physician, who is constantly reminded to be thorough and to act in context. After 24 hours have elapsed and the list has been reformulated, it or elements of it should not thereafter be obliterated or destroyed, but only modified as new evidence accumulates, so that a record of all revisions will be maintained. That is, the subsequent process is wholly supplementary to the original problem list, as it is finally revised.

In the course of a patient's illness, minor episodes arise which the physician may hesitate to define immediately as significant problems on a master problem list. In this situation, the progress note may be titled "temporary problem," and the appropriate symptom or finding (e.g., pain in abdomen) may follow the title. When the time comes for the second progress note to be written, it will be easy to determine whether the temporary problem should be transferred to the problem list or dropped as a transient episode of little significance, not to be referred to again.

In organizations where coding of principal diagnoses is a ritual that can easily be upset by a problem list containing not only diagnoses but physiological and symptomatic findings, those doing the coding need only scan the problem list for the diagnoses. These are always readily apparent to experienced observers. That so many items on problem lists are not diagnoses may seem to be disturbing evidence of our failure to understand completely much of what we deal with, but lack of understanding does not justify omission or neglect in a final tabulation. Indeed, it is precisely on these points, not yet understood and still evolving, that we should continue to focus a critical analysis for the benefit of the patient. Our failure to include such problems in patients' records in the past is evidence of how thoroughly ingrained our episodic approach to medical care is and of how preoccupied we have been with performing medical *tours de force*, as we found solutions to major problems, many of which might have been prevented altogether by a more thoughtful and systematic approach. Physicians must actively develop a capacity and a tolerance for what Whitehead called "sustained muddle-headedness." We must learn to live with ambiguity in the pursuit of honest solutions to difficult problems.

The list of problems should include not only active but inactive or resolved problems (Fig. 5). The latter category includes any previously significant difficulty which may recur or may lead to a complication. For example, removal of a breast, gall bladder surgery, or cholecystitis should always appear on the list. An arm fracture that occurred when the adult patient was a child can be left out completely if, in the opinion of the physician, healing has been complete and no significant future problems can rationally be attributed to it. Disorders such as diabetes or glaucoma should always be considered active problems, regardless of how well controlled they are at the present or how unrelated the current complaint of the patient may seem.

When the physician's time is unavoidably limited, he should not abandon the idea of a complete problem list. Rather he should title the abbreviated list that he is able to formulate "problems not yet completely delineated" and specify the one or two problems he does recognize and proposes to take action on. By labeling the list in this manner he is being completely honest with himself and with all those who depend upon the record. Later, there may be more time. New findings may be made, and the problem list will slowly grow. Honest, accurate notes make all our efforts cumulative, even when we lack time. The nature and extent of any incompleteness is immediately discernible in records containing an honest list of problems and accurately titled progress notes.

In a simple medical situation, such as an appendectomy in a well person, one problem labeled "#1. Appendectomy" and a series of progress notes and plans, each designated #1 and properly titled, will on brief examination tell any physician new to the case that there is a single problem with no complications in an otherwise well person. The student or physician who is the author of the record should immediately be corrected, however, if careful examination of the patient and laboratory data reveals that there are more problems, either not identified or simply neglected. The system is open-ended and allows for the simple and the complex, the ill-defined symptom and the well-established diagnosis. All it requires is that the formulation of problems be explicit to a degree consistent with the current state of their identification and resolution at any point in time.

In those institutions where complete, current problem lists are

```
              ACTIVE PROBLEMS                          INACTIVE PROBLEMS

 #1  Accelerated hypertension

     Retinopathy

     Renal disease

 #2  Hypokalemia—etiology to be
     determined

 #3  Vomiting—dehydration (central
     venous pressure—0, hematocrit 40)

 #4  Diarrhea—unknown etiology

 #5  Anemia, secondary to renal
     disease (Problem #1)

 #6                                             Remote peptic ulcer
                                                disease

 #7                                             Cholecystectomy

 #8  Exogenous obesity

 #9  (L) breast mass

#10                                             History of chronic
                                                alcoholism

#11                                             History of gonorrhea Rx'd

#12                                             Personality disorder

#13  Decreased vision (R) eye
     possible central retinal
     artery occlusion

#14  Cardiac murmur, continuous.
     Never before described ──→
     Chest wall flow murmur second-
     ary to problem #9 (progress
     note 12/4)
```

FIGURE 5. Problem list showing active and inactive (or resolved) problems.

available, they should be enlarged and displayed in the operating room, much as X rays are, so that anesthetists and surgeons are continually reminded that the patient may have far more to contend with than the single difficulty that is monopolizing their attention at the moment. By such a simple technique, nodes that should have been cultured will not be carelessly dropped in formalin, and patients whose cardiovascular status is borderline will not be subjected to lengthy procedures that were hastily decided upon on the basis of a frozen section alone.

In the teaching process, the problem list should be the starting point. The first question should be: Is this list complete? The teacher will know the answer if he is familiar with the case and if he teaches from a data base that he himself has prepared or employed in the past—or from his careful study of the "work-up" of a competent colleague or resident. If the student has defined all the problems, no matter how crudely, then he has reached a minimum standard of thoroughness and reliability with regard to the history-taking and the physical examination. If he has not recognized all of the problems, then a more critical analysis of the student work-up is required. A serious mistake in teaching medicine is to expose the student, the house officer, or the physician to an analytical discussion of the diagnosis and management of one problem before establishing whether or not he is capable of identifying and defining all of the patient's problems at the outset. The approach recommended here teaches more than the technique of obtaining a good history and physical examination. It also teaches the kind of resourcefulness that explores all sources of data, and it inculcates an analytical sense that formulates the data into precisely defined problems that may justly be taken as the foundation of further work. Such an approach emphasizes *process* and *results*, not initial diagnosis that contains elements of assumption and may as a consequence be poorly followed or left unresolved.

When the student lists as separate problems many findings that the experienced physician would recognize as manifestations of a single problem the teacher should immediately recognize that this characteristic defines the level of the student's understanding. Rather than insisting on a premature resolution of the anomalies by ill-advised diagnostic guesswork, the physician-teacher should systematically help the student to synthesize separate clinical symptoms into a valid single entity, just as the physician-teacher, in his bedside teaching, helps the student to analyze a multiplicity of problems.

For the learning physician the problem list can be a source of considerable confusion and an index either to his lack of medical knowledge or of the ability to apply it with thoroughness and precision. The jumbled problem list must be recognized for what it is— a call for help and assistance—the student's clear statement of difficulties that should not be ignored. If it is so recognized, then the problem list may become, for instructor and student alike, the source of progress in knowledge and technique.

PSYCHIATRIC AND DEMOGRAPHIC PROBLEMS

By many physicians, nonorganic problems encountered in the practice of medicine are regarded as alien, baffling, and perhaps not even interesting. Consequently, personality and adjustment problems are usually ignored in summaries of patient problems, even though they could have been described easily using clearly understood non-technical formulations ("cries easily," "family difficulties," etc.) if the physician is unfamiliar with sophisticated psychiatric terminology. Until all psychiatric problems are consistently objects of the physician's attention and have become numbered and titled elements of the problem list, it will not be possible for him to watch them evolve and thereby to learn systematically from his own experience with such problems. Furthermore, by ignoring them he fails to develop his appreciation for patterns of emotional disturbances. His attitude toward modern techniques of analysis may at best be one of perplexity; at worst he may show lack of concern and even rejection.

The computer is making a major contribution in this area. The vast amount of research on the Minnesota Multiphasic Personality Inventory (MMPI) and the computerization of the analyses of the MMPI have made it much more likely, where it is employed, that the patient will gain from his physician an immediate, sympathetic understanding of the forces with which he or she is struggling, and much inadvertent neglect and many inadequate analyses by the medical profession can be avoided. There are many physicians who reject the help of modern techniques on the basis that Osler for three hours followed by Freud for three hours could have done better. Even if this were true, modern techniques are not competing in that league, but rather they are competing with hasty, "off-the-cuff," five-minute analyses by untrained, impatient physicians who live from case to case and who have no systematic means of learning and improving from a highly organized and recorded data base that is kept up to date.

A similar situation exists in regard to problems in demographic medicine. Physicians are still almost exclusively preoccupied with episodic illness. They come to grips with medical problems only when they erupt into symptoms and with patients only when they appear in the office. At the present time it is almost impossible to get a reliable and complete history of illness in a sample of the population or even in an individual. And except for a few pioneers like Robbins and Hall,* most physicians do not even regard demographic problems as continuing concerns, let alone actively seeking to identify, understand, and deal with them. As Robbins and Hall point out, for a forty-year-old woman whose problem list contains only a fractured arm, medicine has completely neglected the major medical significance of the fact that she is forty and female. Over the next ten years her greatest medical risk will be cancer of the breast, and for her a yearly breast examination is the most important part of follow-up therapeutic plans. Physicians are so accustomed to dealing with disease only in the individual and only after it becomes explicit, symptomatic, or terminal that they come by default to believe that medicine is somehow not relevant to health hazards from

* L. C. Robbins, M.D., and J. Hall, M.D., personal communications.

accidents, smoking, diet, smog, stress and social conflict, heredity, obesity, or the simple fact of being forty and male or female. Clearly the problem list should include demographic problems as well as those of other types. References to demographic problems should lead to specific action, appropriately timed, in the interest of prevention or early diagnosis. They should, as well, serve constantly to remind the physician where in health care his total obligations lie.

Paramedical personnel, such as public health workers, social workers, psychologists, and chemists, are already assembling data that make possible the definition of all sorts of social and demographic problems. It is for physicians to assume the leadership in providing each patient with a total list of problems, irrespective of where in the hierarchy of learning the data originated, and in seeing that therapeutic action reflects an adequate perspective on the total needs of the patient.

Those physicians who seek to provide total care for their patients and who naturally integrate findings into well-formulated problem lists should not, and usually do not, feel threatened by the challenge of creating a complete list. The specialist who is annoyed or made anxious when health issues are raised that extend beyond the limited area of his mastery may feel threatened by the strict accounting suggested here. It is certainly true that that accounting sets high and difficult aims, but I suggest that precision in setting and planning for health-care goals cannot ultimately be separated from precision in the practice of our profession. To be blunt: through inefficiency in procuring a broad data base, through failure to keep records properly, and through neglect of quantity of care (even though we point with pride to quality), we physicians have put ourselves in a position in which our capacity to manage rationally or even to define large-scale health-care tasks is in question. To the degree that we are provincial in our understanding of the total health-care job to be done, we should be limited in our power to plan for and control the future of medical practice. To the extent that we are enlightened, we should be allowed to exercise that role.

TWO PROBLEM LISTS

The following problem list, from a general medical ward, is presented here for purposes of study and comment.

#1 Acute encephalopathy
Probably secondary to uremia
Transient anisocoria

#2 Uremia
? Dehydration

#3 Fever
Pyuria without bacteriuria
Leukocytosis

#4 Biventricular congestive failure
Mild

#5 Moth-eaten skull

#6 History adult onset diabetes

#7 Hypertension

#8 Obesity

#9 Dental caries

#10 Abnormal chest X ray

#11 Varicose veins

Our first question should be: Is this list complete? A quick review of the initial data base suggests that it is not; in the first few sentences of the description of the present illness that accompanies this problem list, one reads: "60-year-old white female who (according to her son) was well until 4 AM yesterday when she apparently awoke and was confused, muttering religious phrases, refusing to acknowledge her son's presence. Son denies any fever, chills, seizures, paresis. However, allegedly patient has been vomiting for

2 days." The vomiting is not represented on the list and either should be recorded as a separate problem or should be represented as the first item in problem #2, followed by the presently listed dehydration and uremia, depending upon whether the physician thinks it is possible at the outset to attribute the uremia to this vomiting history.

The next question that should be asked is: Is each problem expressed properly? The first five problems are reviewed one by one below. Each is followed by specific comments relevant to that question.

> #1 Acute encephalopathy
>   Probably secondary to uremia
>   Transient anisocoria

Would acute encephalopathy best be expressed by omitting "probably secondary to uremia"? Unless there is no doubt that the encephalopathy results from uremia, a complete analysis of the problem is in order. Ascribing the encephalopathy to uremia, even "probably," may mislead colleagues and prevent a thorough attack on the problem.

> #2 Uremia
>   ? Dehydration

Question marks should not appear in the problem list. Uremia should simply be worked up and dehydration ruled out (or verified) as one of the causes.

> #3 Fever
>   Pyuria without bacteriuria
>   Leukocytosis

If the physician thinks that the fever is secondary to pyuria, then the problem is simply pyuria, and fever need not be listed. If, on the other hand, he is trying to record the probability that the fever is an independent problem since no bacteriuria exists, then fever should be listed and worked up separately. The plan for a fever of unknown origin is of course quite different from the approach to a fever which is merely secondary to a urinary tract difficulty.

#4 Biventricular congestive failure
   Mild

It should be indicated whether the etiology is unknown or is secondary to problem #7 or some other cause which the physician understands but has failed to mention.

#5 Moth-eaten skull

After reviewing the film, the radiologist objected to this expression, asserting that the film was consistent with hyperparathyroidism.

As the experienced physician studied the amended problem list, his attention would no doubt be drawn to acute encephalopathy, vomiting, uremia, and "pepper and salt" appearance of skull in X ray. He would seek to ascertain the patient's serum calcium. He would not be surprised if it was markedly elevated and would expect this patient at autopsy to have a parathyroid tumor. What about the inexperienced individual? If he rapidly reviewed the differential for each of the problems in a reference text, he would identify the diagnosis or finding that is a common denominator for several of his problems and would arrive at the same conclusion as the senior physician. Thus a disciplined, thorough approach to a set of problems may not only substitute for experience (or intuition) but may be superior to it, because the methodology does not depend on the necessarily limited reach of the mind of one man but permits the mobilization of the experience, and the accurate memory of it, of many experts through the ordinary coupling of a complete list of problems and readily available standard books and articles. "Experience" and "intuition" are words used by many as if their invocation leads to nothing but good. Experience can be incomplete and misleading; intuition can be wrong as well as right, directly relying as it does upon how accurately one interprets the accumulated range of experiences upon which all intuition is based.

The formulation of a problem list like that above, it may be argued, has already been recommended to every clinician and taught to every student. However, auditing of problem lists reveals that many physicians, regardless of intent, do not in practice create or demand thorough and complete problem lists. Nor can it realistically be said that they teach directly from the intern's own problem lists. Frequently teachers deal casually with an eccentric element of the findings, performing feats of synthesis in their own minds of which the house officer or student may be quite unaware. The obvious results may be confusion in patient care and student learning. The intern or house officer should be able to rely on the problem list as the complete superstructure of good patient care. Instructional pyrotechnics, improvisation, and ellipsis are revealed to be defective when the whole transaction between student and teacher is examined. The breadth and detail of the properly prepared problem list leave no gaps for the accidents of ignorance or error, in practice and learning, that irregular approaches inevitably allow.

Our second problem list is also from a general medical ward:

#1 Confusion, etiology unknown

#2 Hypertension, etiology unknown

#3 Psychosomatic abdominal complaints

#4 Urinary tract infection?

#5 Osteo. of spine

#6 Chronic alcoholism

#7 Fever of unknown origin

#8 Metabolic abnormality
    Hyperbilirubinemia

#9 Urinary obstruction, partial

#10 Probable pulmonary edema (see progress note 2/19)*

#11 Hyperkalemia

* This progress note will be found in the last section of Chapter 5, together with comments on this and subsequent progress notes related to this case.

Comments on all but three of the above problems follow.

#1 Confusion, etiology unknown

#2 Hypertension, etiology unknown

The first two problems are concisely and clearly defined, and the experienced physician will quickly be in a position to evaluate the plan for the resolution of these not unusual problems.

#3 Psychosomatic abdominal complaints

This entry stimulates a careful scrutiny of the initial data base. Has the physician mobilized enough symptomatic and objective data to justify defining his problem at this level? If the problem is accepted as it is, the plan will be quite different from the plan that would be developed, for instance, in the case of "abdominal pain, etiology unknown."

#4 Urinary tract infection?

Question marks do not belong on a problem list. Either a urinary tract infection clearly exists or the problems that may suggest that it does should be stated, e.g., specific findings in the sediment, a specific change on an IVP, or a symptom such as dysuria. A logical approach to "working up" any of the latter can be taught; working up a question mark cannot. No scientist should be in the position of guessing what his problem is as he exercises his science. When the problem is originally stated as above, the tendency is to do several urine cultures, to find them negative, and to conclude that the problem is thereby solved, leaving the original complaint, dysuria or frequency, forgotten and unresolved.

The expression "rule out" in a problem list can also trap the physician. For example, if he expresses the problem as "rule out diabetes," he will do a glucose tolerance test, find it normal, and thereby dispose of a difficulty that never existed, leaving the vaginitis or neuropathy buried in some narrative history or physical exam, never to be identified again.

#5 Metabolic abnormality
    Hyperbilirubinemia

"Metabolic abnormality" is meaningless. What is the problem? Is the hyperbilirubinemia the abnormality? If so, the first phrase is redundant. If not, the specific finding should be stated. Also as the hyperbilirubinemia is encountered, the data base must immediately be examined to see why the physician separates the jaundice problem from the chronic alcoholism and how in the face of both of them he can establish with conviction problem #3 as psychosomatic abdominal complaints. As the teacher carefully interrelates a problem list with a data base and progress notes, he can in very specific ways improve the care of the patient and the abstract quality of the performance of the physician.

#9 Urinary obstruction, partial

If problem #4 had been more explicitly stated, it would be much more apparent whether problem #9 should be combined with it into a single, better-defined problem.

#10 Probable pulmonary edema (see progress note 2/19)

The word "probable" should not be used in a problem list. The student (or physician) either knows the patient is suffering from pulmonary edema and should so state the problem, or he should clearly state it in terms of a symptom, or a sign, or an abnormal X ray finding.

4

THE INITIAL PLAN

Plans for the possible diagnosis and management of each problem, keyed by number to the problem list, should be prepared as the next logical step after the problem list has been formulated. *Each problem should have its own plan, numbered correspondingly*, so that an experienced observer can see at a glance whether an anemia, or a urinary tract infection, for example, has a complete and reasonable plan. Too many serious omissions occur when sleeping pills, blood urea nitrogen orders, and side rails are all mixed up in a list of twenty items, which were spun off the top of the physician's head in a totally random fashion. As time goes on, detailed, progressive plans for each problem will appear as a section of the succeeding progress notes (as in the example presented in Fig. 2, Chapter 1). When a well-conceived plan is written at the outset, all that is necessary for long periods in the progress notes is a record of the data as they are produced. The initial statement of plans is important because it establishes the character of the further data that are to be obtained and the treatment that is to be given.

The patient profile and complete list of problems should be re-examined before plans are prepared for any single problem. Awareness of the patient's way of life and of the whole range of his problems is essential in the avoidance of surgery and medical treatments that may be disastrous in a given context, though they are indicated for a particular problem in isolation. Through a more thorough awareness of the patient's milieu, the physician is in a better position to help him establish or modify personal objectives—with regard, for instance, to returning to work, caring for children, or entering a nursing home.

Obviously, the physician should not endanger an over-all objective in order to pursue the "ideal" resolution or management of a single problem. Moreover, he must strive for a clear idea of what the norm is for a given patient in a given age group before plans are conceived, though it is unfortunately true that in many instances the physician cannot be provided with sharply defined standards when setting goals, either in diagnosis or management. All classification systems and programs for management are arbitrary. There is not a standard case of lupus or angina or emphysema or depression; nor is there an absolute amount of insulin or fluid or bicarbonate for a patient with diabetic acidosis. But there are variables prominently associated with each disorder and its management. If each variable is identified and restored to, or maintained in, a normal state, and the physician thinks more in terms of logical biochemistry, physiology, and psychology than in terms of artificially conceived syndromes and categories, then he is less likely to be frustrated and misled by what may be referred to as polemics in medicine.

In taking a physiological approach to a patient's difficulties, we physicians must continually remind ourselves of how little of the total picture we are able to see, particularly in the first encounter with a patient. In general, if a patient has developed complicated difficulties over a course of weeks or months, we should not try to extricate him from those difficulties in minutes with an eccentric therapy that is directed only to the derangements readily apparent. Thoughtless, over-rapid readjustment of a few parameters, considered out of context, can be dangerous to the patient.

It is true that prognosis requires diagnosis, but diagnosis always leads to a degree of categorization that is never wholly justified. Physicians must learn for themselves—and teach their patients—a certain measure of planned ambiguity. Otherwise they will make absolute statements, draw premature conclusions, and neglect to follow carefully the progress of the patient, thereby failing in turn to introduce the critical control and continuing readjustment that good medicine always requires. The parameters to which the physician chooses to pay continuing attention are the most important part of any plan, for such follow-up is the only protection the patient has against our misconceptions as we diagnose, treat, and prognosticate. Patients must come to think of a physician as a sophisticated guidance system and not as an oracle with absolute and immediate answers.

Specific plans should be delineated for each problem separately (as in Fig. 6.) They fall into three categories: (1) plans for collection of further data in order to establish a diagnosis or facilitate management; (2) plans for treatment with specific procedures or drugs; and (3) plans for education of the patient about his illness and his part in managing it.

In the preceding chapter it was established as a principle that the expressions "rule out" or "probable" should not be employed in the problem list (though in conventional medical record-keeping such diagnostic guesses are not uncommon). To "rule out" is a diagnostic plan, not a problem, and falls logically under the first of the categories mentioned above. "Probable" also is a signal that further data should be obtained. If the diagnosis is already known and further information is required for skillful management, general statements should be avoided and specific parameters to be followed in a progress note or on a flow sheet (Chapters 5 and 6) should be identified instead, with an indication of the frequency with which they should be obtained.

Many students find it difficult to separate diagnostic activities from those undertaken for immediate therapeutic action. For example, when a patient is in shock, the physician should first think physiologically. He should obtain information about volume, cardiac output, and peripheral resistance and act immediately. He should then systematically procure information to determine the cause. To say that in life-threatening situations one must determine the cause

```
                        Problem List

        #1.  Failure to thrive, etiology unknown

        #2.  RUQ mass questionable

        #3.  Glanular  hypospadius, congenital

Plan

#1.  Failure to thrive, etiology unknown

    a.  R.O.  Environmental deprivation

             Start feedings with Formula #2, 100cc/kgm, i.e., 50-60 cc q4h

    b.  R.O.  Cardiovascular etiology

             Chest film

    c.  R.O.  Renal etiology

             Urinanalysis:  RFT—BUN, creatinine

             Urine culture

             IVP

    d.  R.O.  Gastrointestinal etiology

             Stool examination for pH, reducing substances, fat, occult blood

             Serum carotene levels

             Consider UGI series with follow through
```

FIGURE 6. Initial plan for a three-problem pediatric problem list. The plan has not been edited. Abbreviations are as follows:

BUN = blood urea nitrogen	PBI = protein-bound iodine
CBC = complete blood count	RFT = renal function tests
CID = cytomegalic inclusion disease	R.O. = rule out
	r/o = rule out
CNS = central nervous system	RUQ = right upper quadrant
GU = genitourinary	STS = serological tests for syphilis
IVP = intravenous pyelogram	
q4h = every four hours	UGI = upper gastrointestinal

        e.   R.O.   Metabolic etiology

                     Ca. phos, alk, phos

                     Urinary amino acids

        f.   R.O.   CNS

                     Transillumination of skull

                     Serum titers for CID, rubella, toxoplasma

                     STS

        g.   R.O.   Hematological etiology
                     CBC

                     Blood smear

        h.   R.O.   Endocrine etiology

                     Electrolytes, r/o Addison's

                     PBI, r/o hypothyroidism

        i.   R.O.   Milk allergy syndromes

                     Change formula to nutramigen

#2.   RUQ mass, questionable

       Urinanalysis

       Flat plate and upright

       IVP

#3.   Glanular hypospadius, congenital

                IVP to r/o obstruction

                GU consult

FIGURE 6 (Continued)

before taking action is like saying that we must know why the child fell in the water before we will take steps to retrieve him. It is customary to take adaptive and contingency actions to satisfy immediate needs; therefore the physician is rarely justified in prematurely assigning causes before a reasonable body of facts is available.

When it is necessary to acquire diagnostic information over an extended period of time, it becomes difficult for physicians to think etiologically in a sustained and organized manner, especially after immediate physiological disturbances have been corrected. There is a great tendency to think vigorously about causes at the time of admission and then to fall into an uncritical attitude as day-to-day details are managed and the preponderance of the physician's energies are turned to new admissions. It is therefore essential that the initial plan be given much thought and that problem-oriented progress notes, with supplemental plans, be so kept that over-all execution can be judged and reassessments made without confusion. In complex cases the emphasis should be on quick daily review of each active problem to ensure that a maximum effort is being exerted to resolve it, as opposed to an aimless collection of further information of questionable utility.

In the second category (plans for treatment with drugs or procedures), plans should be specific; entries such as "postural drainage" or "fluids" or "antibiotics" are insufficient because they are general and uninformative.

The third category (plans for education of the patient) has been seriously neglected by the medical profession. When patients are discharged, the physician fully expects that they will understand and manage their own procedures and drugs and diets, when in reality they may often be wholly confused, not only about the character of the treatment but also about the function of it and about what effect a particular drug is supposed to produce or a particular personal regimen is intended to create. In the last analysis, the patient with a chronic disease must in large part be his own physician; if he does not understand his own illness and its treatment, moments of reprimand and irritability in the office of the busy practitioner or busy clinic will provide little in the way of correctives. It is not surprising that studies of compliance in medical therapy indicate a level of noncompliance as high as 25 to 50 per cent.

Many physicians are inclined to believe it unnecessary specifically to plan the education of the patient (and when I speak of patient education I refer not only to therapeutic directions but to the whole range of information that is imparted to the patient about his illness). They rely on the improvisation of the moment, and in so doing they slight the importance of this third category and, what is more, by keeping no problem-oriented record of what in fact has been said tó the patient about his illness they run the serious risk of omission or contradiction. Concise phrases, in the telegraphic style of the remainder of the plan, are perfectly appropriate for inclusion in category three; they will be sufficient to establish the framework of the dialogue with the patient and so to indicate when the expectations the physician has created have been unfulfilled, to permit the readjustment of the information given the patient in the light of the developing medical situation, and to ensure the full mobilization of his respect and confidence. If the problem is a recurrence of a duodenal ulcer, perhaps the third category under the corresponding plan will note, "Patient told he can control with diets and meds as before." That brief entry may be an invaluable reminder at a later date if control by diet and medications, contrary to the physician's expectations, is not successful and the patient must abruptly be asked to accept surgery. Indeed, it may be observed that the patient can sometimes draw an immeasurable reassurance from the simple acknowledgment by the physician of necessary contradiction.*

Physicians should keep in mind that their professional proficiency is the result of a repetition of basic concepts and principles through many years of medical school and residency training. They should not expect the patient to grasp, after one exposure, all the implications and details of the management of his disorder. Indeed, if we dismissed students from medical school or physicians from training on the same standards of learning that some doctors apply

* A particularly useful reference on the subject of patient education is H, Winter Griffith, *Instructions for Patients*, Philadelphia, W. B. Saunders, 1968.

to their patients ("they just don't understand"), I venture to say that there would be few doctors left in the system. As a doctor learns best through his own work and his own progress notes, if carefully led and observed, so does a patient learn best from his own experiences, when carefully led and observed by his physician. Present patients and potential patients are the largest untapped resource in medical care today. Advantage can be taken of that resource through education of the patient and through clear formulation of the role that patients themselves can play as effective paramedical personnel.

5

THE PROGRESS NOTES

The uncertainties inherent in complex biologic systems make properly titled and numbered progress notes the most crucial part of the medical record. They are the mechanism of follow-up on each problem. (Appendix E and Figure 7 will serve as illustrations of clear, orderly, well-prepared progress notes.) Faulty understanding and defective decisions may be expected at the outset of a new case. Indeed, they are inevitable in the face of multiple variables. But failure to follow up rigorously the results of those decisions is inexcusable. Action without follow-up is arrogance, especially where the objects of that action are living systems about which nothing is completely understood and in which conditions never remain fixed.

The progress notes should be written in a form which relates them unmistakably to the problem. Each note should be preceded by the number and title of the appropriate problem. This method immediately tells the reader that it is the progress of anemia (or the urinary tract infection, etc.) that is the subject under discussion. If a new problem is being discussed, it should be added to the original list and dated and numbered accordingly. No progress note should be written without attention being paid to previous progress notes on the same problem.

As can be seen from Fig. 7, each problem-oriented section of the progress note may consist of any or all of the following elements:

Subjective data (headed *Subj*—or *Sx*, for symptomatic data)

Objective data (headed *Obj*)

Interpretation (headed *Imp*, for impressions)

Treatment and therapy (headed *Rx*)

Immediate plans (headed *Plan*)

Additional elements are sometimes added with self-explanatory headings (e.g., *Disc* in Fig. 7, *Negs* in Fig. 4 in Chapter 2). When the physician moves within this framework, his ability to choose the important parameters to be followed, his standards of logic, and his sense of responsibility in the attack upon and resolution of the patient's problems can immediately be appreciated. In addition, as the physician selects certain problems to work on, he reveals which ones he thinks important and, conversely, reveals precisely what he chooses to ignore.

Each of the five elements listed above is commented on below.

SUBJECTIVE DATA. This element includes all the subjective information, including symptomatic data, and is always placed first to ensure that the patient's point of view will be taken into consideration at the outset—a consideration that is seriously neglected by many physicians, who tend to emphasize laboratory and X ray results. Assigning symptomatic data priority in the progress note goes a long way toward correcting that neglect. Valuable information available in no other way can be derived from the patient's symptomatology.

OBJECTIVE DATA. In the objective data section of the progress note, doctors are frequently inclined to omit valuable physical findings that should be included. For example, a white count, chest X ray, or sputum culture may be recorded as objective data in the note on a pulmonary problem without any mention of the patient's physical signs or of the character and quality of his sputum production.

#1. Failure to thrive

    <u>Subj</u>: Patient in no distress, feeding well

    <u>Obj</u>: PE: T = 37.3

          HR = 140/min

          RR = 28/min

          Otherwise unchanged

          CXR: no infiltrate, no cardiomegaly

          Weight: up 150 gm after two days of formula #2

    <u>Rx</u>: None

    <u>Imp</u>: Thriving well on present diet.

    <u>Plan</u>: 1. observe and maintain on present formula.

#2. RUQ mass, questionable

    <u>Subj</u>: None

    <u>Obj</u>: PE: abd.—the RUQ mass can no longer be palpated with certainty.

          Flat plate and upright: no masses or fluid levels

          UA: negative, except s.g. = 1.007

          Urine culture: negative

          RFT: BUN = 26; Creatinine = 0.6

    <u>Rx</u>: None

    <u>Disc</u>: Although original RUQ mass not supported by any of the studies

          so far obtained, the possibility of a neuroblastoma or Wilm's

          tumor cannot be ruled out on flat plate. Thus will do IVP.

    <u>Imp</u>: Probably no RUQ mass

    <u>Plan</u>: 1. Schedule IVP

FIGURE 7. Problem-oriented progress notes. This unedited series of notes was made in connection with the pediatric case whose problem list and initial plans are given

1/6

#2. RUQ mass, questionable

   Obj: IVP: bilateral prompt excretion of dye, without evidence for

       caliceal blunting or ureteral dilitation. No caliceal dis-

       placement or distortion.

   Imp: No renal etiology for RUQ mass

   Plan: 1. Drop diagnosis

1/8

#1. Failure to thrive

   Subj: Still feeding well, in no distress

   Obj: Afebrile

      PE: no change

      Weight: no gain since 1/5

   Disc: Appears that environmental factors not significant in this

       patient's failure to thrive, since no weight gain on good

       intake. Neoplasm as an etiology ruled out—see problem #2

       —1/6. GI causes should be ruled out next.

   Imp: Etiology still unclear

   Plan: 1. Change formula to nutramigen

       2. Stool work-up—see original impressions 1: plan 6

FIGURE 7 (Continued)

in Fig. 6. Abbreviations not included in the caption to Fig. 6 are:

CXR = chest X ray	Imp = impressions	RR = respiratory rate
Disc = discussion	(interpretation)	Rx = treatment and therapy
HR = heart rate	Obj = objective data	Sub = subjective data
	PE = physical examination	UA = urinalysis

Noting perhaps that a respirator was used, the doctor too often omits any note of routines being applied to help the patient with coughing and drainage, or even the patient's ability to cooperate. In those problems that require the creation of a flow sheet (as described in the next chapter), the doctor simply enters "see flow sheet" in the objective data section of the progress note.

INTERPRETATION. In the interpretive (or "impressions") section of the progress note, physicians should keep in mind the original plan and objectives. Also, when disagreements arise, for example on the subject of whether surgery should be employed in an elderly patient with a number of problems, the progress notes should contain written evidence that expert consultants, representing both sides of the issue, personally met, discussed the matter, and reached a conclusion. Unilateral action is practically never necessary if systematic approaches to difficult situations are formulated and followed.

TREATMENT AND THERAPY. A significant modification in therapy or diagnostic action should never be made without careful reference to previous progress notes on the same problem. Frequently, earlier evidence, however unassailable, is neither supported nor refuted; it is never interpreted or even appreciated. It is ignored. Often these data were obtained at great discomfort and expense to the patient and, if studied, may provide the evidence needed to solve the patient's current problems.

IMMEDIATE PLANS. The "plan" section of the progress note, like the initial plan, should be prepared not only with respect to the specific problem but to other problems as well, so that therapy which ordinarily would be satisfactory will be withheld when contraindicated by other problems noted in the complete list. As soon as modifications or additions to the initial plans are indicated, the notes should state these clearly.

Organization of progress notes in the above manner continually reminds the physician to think systematically about a patient and provides evidence of whether he has actually done so. The younger physician will develop a pattern of ideation for each type of problem and will thereby create a framework upon which to build his postgraduate self-education.

Nurses' notes, social service notes, and physical medicine notes should not be separate parts of a medical record but should themselves be progress notes of the kind recommended here, properly titled with respect to specific problems and placed in sequence with all other data pertaining to a given problem. In this manner the medical and paramedical professions assume an integrated and easily audited role in solving the patient's problems, and each avoids establishing the kind of identity that permits or encourages the possibility of dealing with problems out of context. It serves an educational function for every nurse and social worker to review constantly the total problem list and to enter all observations and actions under the appropriate heading; understanding (or the lack thereof) is immediately revealed when such entries are associated with the appropriate (or inappropriate) problem.

When paramedical findings suggest difficulties not yet identified in the problem list, it is the obligation of paramedical personnel to define a new problem or to call to the attention of the physician the necessity of doing so. In family clinics the record of the head of the household should contain copies of the problem lists of all members of his household for the physician's quick perusal, so that he will not be inclined to reach contextually unrealistic decisions or make contextually unrealistic recommendations.

RESIDENT NOTES

The approaches to the medical record described here can do much to define the role and the responsibilities of the resident physician. The conventional extended note of the resident is no longer recommended. Instead, after he has "worked up" his patient he should review and correct where necessary the list of problems as defined by the intern. The resident must first ascertain whether all the problems have been identified. He should critically examine the historical, physical, and laboratory evidence that bears on each.

He should then insert after each problem an entry that consists of either "agree" or of a specific amendment.

The resident should use the problem list as the focus for work rounds and the implementation of complete day-to-day care. He should insist that the list of problems be complete and current and that the level of resolution of each problem be apparent. A good resident rapidly learns what problems should be given priority and naturally refrains from casual discussion of complex issues without carefully reading the appropriate problem-oriented progress notes and flow sheets.

A resident can measure his progress as a teacher and leader, not by how extensive his notes of amendment are but by how brief, and by how infrequently it is necessary for him to reformulate the list of problems. If an intern fails to develop under a given resident, then documentation of this failure, explicit in the medical record, and particularly in the resident's notes, should be made available to the faculty, preferably by the resident himself. When house officers, students, and practicing physicians are evaluated in any other manner, interpersonal factors irrelevant to their capacity to care effectively for patients may intrude. The more tightly coupled care and education become by means of the medical record, the more secure are the welfare of the patient and the rights of the physician in charge of his care.

OPERATIVE NOTES

Operative notes are elements in the record of the patient's progress and should always appear as numbered and titled entries in the progress notes. If operative findings throw new light on the definition of problems, the problem list should be modified accordingly:

#1. Abdominal Pain → Carcinoma of the pancreas [Date of finding]

Complications following surgery should be stated as new problems, followed by the entry "secondary to problem # [the original problem]." Data on a series of complications, such as pneumonia, phlebitis, fistulas, and the like, should not be consolidated into a single note because of the confusion that would result.

At the time the surgeon writes the operative note he should quickly review the complete problem list, stating under the appropriate number in a titled progress note whether additional useful information about a kidney or a liver, for example, became available at surgery. No opportunity should ever be lost to add significant data to the medical record.

CONSULTANT NOTES

The consultant will of course examine the patient and the data in the customary manner. He will be expected, however, to enter his note in a form that differs significantly from that usually observed in most medical records, in which known facts are intermingled with new information and conclusions are buried in pages of narrative.

A consultant should identify the problem for which he was consulted. He should employ its proper number and title and immediately state in not more than a line or two his conclusions and principal recommendations. He should then, under a separate subentry entitled *Discussion*, defend the position he has taken, repeating data already recorded in the chart only as they are employed analytically to support his conclusions.

Having completed this annotation, he should then review the problem list, adding any new problems that may have been revealed and recording under the appropriate problem number and title any new information or additional analysis that his specialized point of view contributes. When he has nothing significant to record with regard to a specific problem, he of course omits mention of it. If this approach is taken and if all the data on any given problem are retrieved in sequence, all relevant contributions are immediately available in context to the primary physician and others. At the present time, many specialists either do not consider all the patient's problems and so provide a stereotyped analysis rather than one tailored to the patient's peculiar range of difficulties or, if they do approach the totality of the patient's problems, do not integrate their own analysis with the ongoing analysis by the physician in charge of the patient. If the specialist cannot use the existing list because he thinks it is incomplete or inadequately expressed, his first order of business should be to discuss it with the physician in charge; otherwise his note may be ignored as a fragment never fully integrated into the ongoing appraisal of patient needs.

CRITIQUE OF A PROGRESS NOTE

The progress note that follows relates to the second of the two problem lists that were discussed in detail at the end of Chapter 3. The complete problem list will be found there. We are concerned here only with problems #1, #7, and #10.

Progress Note 2/9*

#7 Fever of Unknown Origin

> Sx: None (specific)
>
> Obj: This AM the patient spiked a T of 41°
>
> RR = 36–48 min BP 200/160 —
>
> ↑ 130/80
>
> Lung rales at bases—rhonchi diffusely throughout
>
> Chest X ray—no localized infiltrate
>
> Gm stain sputum: gm + cocci
>
> Gm stain urine: gm - encap. rods. Probable Klebsiella
>
> Imp: Prob. gm - sepsis
>
> Plan: 1. Cultures blood, urine
>
> 2. Ice blanket
>
> 3. Rx pen. Kana + colistin

---

* Abbreviations used in this progress note are as follows:

BP = blood pressure	pen = penicillin
Dx = diagnosis	RR = respiratory rate
CXR = chest X ray	SOB = short of breath
H.R. = heart rate	Sx = subective data
hr = hour	T = temperature

#1 Confusion

    Sx: Completely obtunded today—unresponsive

    Obj: Neck rigid

           Neuro exam unchanged

    Imp: ? Secondary to intracranial bleeding

    Plan: Will not do spinal tap now

           Other problems more important

In any patient with single or multiple unexplained findings or problems, each should be pursued to its logical conclusion. Often when this is done, synthesis of several problems into a single entity occurs as a natural consequence of thoroughness of exploration and application of simple logic. For example, had a lumbar puncture been done and pus found, problem #7 as well as #1 might have been far less obscure. Accurate, complete information is the foundation of good management, and it is ultimately economical of time to obtain it rather than to attempt to improvise without it.

#10 Probable pulmonary edema

    Sx: As above

    Obj: BP falling → 160/90

           Hr 160/min

           RR 36–48/min

           Patient suddenly developed acute SOB + frothing at mouth. ?Pulm. edema

    Imp: Pulm. edema

    Plan: Rx dig., morph. + phlebotomy 150cc

           CXR—did not confirm

           No diuretics because of possible gm neg. sepsis

Many elements of these progress notes suggest the physician is inexperienced and unsure of himself, but this useful observation could not so readily be made if he had not titled his notes and grouped his facts and interpretations accordingly. Without the titles, the incongruity, incompleteness, and faulty analysis might well have been overlooked in the review of the notes.

When the progress note is read by the resident or attending physician for the purpose of guiding the intern, the critique should be presented in an orderly manner. First the title: If "probable" indicates that the intern wasn't sure of his entry, why did not the title reflect what he was sure of—in this case the findings? The resident or teacher should sit down with the intern and actually prepare a note that is more appropriate under the circumstances. Such a note should not be entered into the record but is intended instead as an example from which the intern may learn. For instance:

#10 Acute fall in BP, tachypnea, and tachycardia

> *Sx:*   Unresponsive
>
> *Obj:*   See #7—particularly chest findings and chest film (should make time relationship to physical findings clear).
> BP now 160/90
> H.R. 160/min
> "Frothing at mouth"
> Chest exam—see above
>
> *Imp:*   Except for "frothing" not picture of pulmonary edema (if rales only at bases)
> BP fall, tachypnea and tachycardia consistent with pulmonary embolism or with septicemia as discussed under #7, or infarct
>
> *Plan:*   a. R.O. pulmonary embolus; EKG for typical change, enzymes, *call resident* about further emergency studies.
> R.O. pulmonary edema suggested by "frothing."
> R.O. myocardial infarct—EKG
> b. Consult resident about instituting morphine. phlebotomy and digitalis, even though Dx much in doubt.
> c. No entry for patient education.

Titled progress notes should be consulted at autopsy so that the findings may be correlated as precisely as possible with the perceptions of the physician as he progressively identified and analyzed problems. (This patient underwent another episode in which the blood pressure fell to 90 and at autopsy showed massive pulmonary emboli.) The original physician should be asked to discuss exactly what was meant by "frothing at the mouth," since that factor played a major role in his conclusion.

With regard to patients such as the one described here, the teacher can be very explicit about the occasions on which the intern should request assistance. Whenever the physician is uncertain and is able to define his problem merely in terms of findings that suggest that the patient is in danger, he should get help. That help was obtained should be reflected in the patient's record, either as a note by the resident or teacher or a direct quote of his advice. A call for the right help at the right time is often the most intelligent part of a good plan.

New house officers rotating into difficult general medical services from specialty services are suddenly confronted with enormous responsibilities that are well beyond their experience and that require more time for careful consideration than is likely to be available. If they will cooperate in revealing the structure of their thinking to the extent that this house officer did, they will be guided in a manner that is sufficiently relevant for intellectual growth to occur. Naturally, to be intelligible may mean to be found out, and the physician may sometimes wonder whether he ought to be explicit if he thereby makes himself so vulnerable to rigorous analysis. But it is this explicitness and vulnerability that lead to sound education, and that, above all, is what he is after.

6

FLOW SHEETS

For certain problems progress notes are not an adequate means of relating multiple variables. Data involving physical findings, vital signs, laboratory values, medications, and intakes and outputs can lead to sound interpretations and decisions only if they are organized to reveal temporal relationships clearly. Too often younger physicians may observe that the senior physician is likely to scan a patient record, expound on a single laboratory value, call at random for others in an expressionistic way, and finish by reaching doubtful conclusions, prefaced perhaps by the phrase, "in my experience." Time relations are ignored, crucial data are never brought to light, and wrong decisions forever go unrecognized because no logical tracks are discernible in the randomly recorded data.

Flow sheets like those reproduced at the end of this chapter can be used to facilitate the comprehension and interpretation of interrelated and changing variables. On certain fast-moving problems, the flow sheet may constitute the only progress note. The time required initially in setting up a proper flow sheet is small compared to that lost in unraveling and reassembling disorganized and misplaced data.

In the construction of flow sheets, basic principles should be emphasized to the student at once. The teacher should spend more time helping the student decide what parameters to follow and how frequently to follow them and less time predicting conclusions. The data will tell the young physician what to do, but he needs help in acquiring the discipline to keep his information orderly and to audit it systematically.

In choosing the appropriate parameters to follow for a given problem, the physician should keep in mind that he must strike a balance between an excessive number of variables and a compulsive preoccupation with the precision of a single variable, which, if interpreted by itself, could be very misleading. For example, the determination of four or five variables of a completely different type with speed and reasonable accuracy will solve an anemia problem faster than the investment of expensive time in procuring one determination of a single variable to an unreasonable precision or at a frequency that is physiologically absurd. This principle applies to narrative as well as numeric information. The limited time of the physician should not be spent disproportionately on qualifying and quantifying a single term like hemoptysis, if no time is left to resolve the problem by exploring other questions and obtaining and making use of physical findings and a chest X ray.

The frequency of record-keeping (or data collecting) depends upon "how steep the curve is." A chart of a rapidly changing burn patient might show recordings every hour, whereas a chart on a patient with cirrhosis and persistent ascites might show recordings once a week, or once a month. The frequency should be such that the configuration of the patient's course can be detected at a glance.

The bulk of the rapidly moving problems that require a flow sheet are so-called fluid balance problems, and fortunately a few fundamental parameters common to all of them can be emphasized. For example, all patients being maintained on intravenous fluids and patients with renal failure, cardiac failure, shock, acute intestinal problems requiring fluids and drainage, and acidosis—either metabolic or respiratory—require the same careful consideration of the total volume of fluid in the body, of the circulating volume, of the tonicity of fluids, of the potassium level, and of the pH of the fluids. If the student is told to follow the patient's blood pressure, pulse, respiration, venous pressure (by physical examination alone when indicated), hematocrit, and weight, he will almost invariably mobilize his own common sense, make intelligent decisions about volume, and so prevent either the overloading or the "work-up" dehydration that occurs on medical and surgical services. Matters should of course not be allowed to proceed to the point that gross symptoms and physical findings are necessary to alert the physician. If he is told to watch the serum sodium, he will not create or ignore significant derangements in body tonicity. He should carefully watch the serum potassium and the factors like pH that affect it, and he will gradually, from his own flow sheets, gain understanding and pursue the relevant literature as his cases require it. The same is true where pH and blood urea nitrogen are the prime factors.

Having become disciplined about these few parameters common to many problems, the student will quickly learn to add the more specific ones, such as pCO$_2$ and minute-ventilation in the respiratory problem or a series of EKG strips and medications in a patient with a hypertensive crisis or an arrhythmia.

The important point is always to keep from inundating the student or intern with information when what he needs, over and over again, is the opportunity to see principles operating naturally in his own patient as he lines up, side by side and day by day, all the related parameters. If teachers looked more carefully at flow sheets with students, pointed out missing parameters, and directed reading to very specified points, they would misinform less and inculcate discipline more—and learn a great deal themselves.

PROBLEM LIST

#1. Arteriosclerotic heart disease

#2. Seizure disorder ? etiology

#3. Irreversible shock

#4. Pernicious anemia—doubt

#5. Diabetes mellitus

#6. Status post cholecystectomy

#7. Hepatomegaly

#8. Azotemia

#9. Mild dehydration

This single flow sheet offers an excellent opportunity to discuss many aspects of the shock problem. Parameters that deal with volume and cardiac output and indirectly with peripheral resistance are all present, and the quality of care can be assessed with respect to some of the finest details. If an experienced observer feels that certain other parameters should have been followed, he should point them out to the student so that he may add them to the next flow sheet and literally feel himself develop in the management of difficult problems such as this.

Date: ....
Name: W. Q.

Date / Time	BP	P/RR	Wt	CVP	Hct	Arterial pH	pCO₂	O₂ Sat	Na/K	Venous pH	pCO₂	O₂ Sat	In / Out		Notes
2/12 9PM	100/90	80/24	52.1	–	48	7.34	53.1	91%	123/4.3	–	–	–	1675	+740 ml	
2/13 2PM	0/0	80/40	53.4	290	51	7.11	80.5	93%	125/6.6	BUN-49	1.02	63	34%	50cc NaHCO₃ / 450cc D₅W	Coma
3PM	0/0	88/44	–	322						O₂Δ vol% 11				500cc Blood	Coma
4AM	0/0	Intubat 80/80	–	370	41	7.15	26.5	97%		1.02	50	52%	50cc NaHCO₃ / 250cc	3:15 Coma
5PM	100/98	78	196		39	124	32	77%		O₂Δ vol% 7.5		53%	50cc NaHCO₃ / 250	Begins to respond to words
5:30	80/78	158							108/4.8				50K NaHCO₃ 980	Skin warmer
7:30	110/100	80	190										50cc Na 45	
8:15	100/32	180							124/5.1/5.2	BUN-49	53	72%	SS Na/D₅W 1020 / SS 1080	
10:25	100/111	178			39	7.29	50	95%	126/5.0	BUN-49 O₂Δ -3.4	7.28	48	75%	50cc Na / 30 / D₅W 1110	Sleeping but arousable
WT1	88/28	180			36	7.32	50	95%		O₂Δ 4.0			1140	1000 D₅W	
2AM	80/32	160											Na 30 / 18cc	
3AM	70/28	160											1600 SS0	
WT	56/34	148											550 SS / 13cc	Opens eyes on command
WT	70	174				7.31	44	96%	7.05-5.13	Δ 7.49	44	69%	50K Na / 108	

PROBLEM LIST

#1. Acute respiratory insufficiency
    —Acute CO_2 retention
    —Respiratory acidosis

#2. Chronic restrictive and obstructive lung disease
    —(L) pneumonectomy

#3. Trilobar pneumonia

#4. Thyromegaly

#5. Acute cor pulmonale with right ventricular failure

#6. Pulmonary tuberculosis—inactive

It is apparent from this flow sheet and list of problems that this patient was desperately ill with pneumonia throughout her only lung, with a pH of 6.94, a pCO_2 of greater than 150 and an oxygen saturation of 85 per cent, when she was receiving oxygen before the intubation and subsequent tracheostomy. With all the parameters (including the minute ventilation), recorded at the time by the intern in a routine ward, one has no better vehicle than the flow sheet for the presentation of the principles of respiratory physiology and total care.

DATE TIME	B.P.	P/R	T	V.P.	Wgt.	Hct	Na	CO2	pH	O2	O2 MIN	SH HCO3	I-V O/I	INPUT OUTPUT urine	MEDS & PROCEDURES
5-27 6 PM	174/120	117/36	7/30		62/132	5.2	27.5	6.94		65.72	4 min				① Start O₂ - Intubation done with Bird Respirator ② Venisection - Removed 500 cc
6³⁰ PM	180/90	108							7/30						
7⁰⁰ PM									7.05 / 12³	96.7	3.4				←10 m. morphine 30y no respirations without Bird Depressive
8 PM	116/96	104	36.°	21							3.8	500 / 0.5			← Amphy/dopa 250 mg I-V own
9⁰⁰ PM		104/90	9³ᵉʳ					6.97 / 7.45			3.6	500 / 0.5			9 om 6 ₁ₘ 176 meq K⁺ HCO₃⁻
10 PM	130/70	96/9						7.11 / 7.40		98.7%	3.8	500 / 1.1	0.5 / Hicont large amt		
11 PM	110/70	108/9	15	50				7.13 / 7.06	8.1°		4.7				11 AM 2990 I-V 11.30 11.30 TRACHEOSTOMY PERFORMED
5-28 12³⁰ AM	94/60	110/9						7.33 / 7.5	14°		3.6		0.5 / Hicont large amt		
2 AM	130/70	94/9									3.3				3 AM Responding to painful stimulations
4 AM	74/44	74/9	9												
6 AM	84/48	101/10	25	50				8.6 / 7.13	9.36	4.0	150 / 1170	600 / 6°°		Blood Gas 4 hrs. CTE	
9 AM	90.09	108/41	72			67/72	135	28 / 4.7	7.12			0.5 / 1200			230 cc of Blood Removed Venisection 0.25 neg. I-V.
12 noon	87/83	107/11					132	131		4.0	1700				neg. I-V. 0.25 neg. I-V. 0.160 neg. I-V.
5 PM	119/108	129	22.5			67/87	131		7.49				1200 / 900		I.V.

Medical flow sheet (handwritten, rotated)

MK

DATE Time	BP	P/R	T	H.P. Ngt.	Hct /BUN	Na /K	CO2 /Cl	pH /pCO2	pO2 /pO2 sat	min mnt	BH HCO3	I.V /T	INPUT-OUTPUT /T Urine	Notes
5-4 8 AM	162/114	100/16	37.6	59.6	44/9	14°/44	45	7.34/96	45	3.7	39	1300/3200	320/0-5	WBC 7500
10	154/100	90/9	38.7		45/5	143/16	445	7.34/122	98	3.2	36		1700	
PM													1200	
5-30	148/44	112/47	57.6	45/7	144/7	45/-	7/222	135 p.o.			222/3170		* ON THE BIRD RESPIRATOR
5-31	130/86	.001/16	55.5	42/7	141/7	49/90	7.35/238	198/200*			1700	1300	251/	
6-1			55.6									2445	1200	
6-2	138/78	96/	51.9	42/7	144/8	48/90	7.2/162	49/142			2510	1800	
6-3	140/90	100/	50.7	42/7		36/45					1870	835	
6-4	141/86	90/	44.7			36/35						475	
6-5	136/80	80/	50.7			48	10/	200			1760	715	
6-6	124/74	88/	44.69	42/8	42/8		121/151	122/180			2370		
6-7	130/90	90/10	51.0	44/11	44/9								URINE pH = 8.0
6-13	130/80	90/12					52.2/5.5	123/49 4.9/49***	89				*** OFF THE BIRD WITH TRACHEOTOMY — PLUGGED
6-22	130/44	44/12	51.6	44/									

PROBLEM LIST

#1. Paroxysmal atrial tachycardia

#2. Acute pneumonitis—bacterial

#3. Chronic obstructive lung disease—acute asthma

#4. Hepatomegaly

#5. Calcific pericarditis, status post-op pericardial stripping

#6. Calcific pleuritis

#7. Stasis dermatitis—legs

#8. Acute myocardial infarction 11/17

#9. Diabetes mellitus—adult onset 11/19

This flow sheet on an arrhythmia problem reveals to the student or house officer how difficult it is to draw conclusions about drugs when four or five agents are used in rapid succession. With data such as this available, one does not easily fall in the trap of saying (and believing), "I had a patient yesterday with an interesting arrhythmia which we handled with Dilantin."

Also one should note that, although the problem list includes chronic lung disease, no pH, pCO_2, or O_2 saturation are on the flow sheets as appropriate parameters to be watched while the attempt is made to control the cardiac rhythm. Drugs such as Dilantin cannot overcome the wrong metabolic environment in which the heart is trying to function. Also there is no column in which the sedation can be carefully followed.

DATE: 11-13-65
NAME:

Date/Time	EKG Strip (II ɑ AVF)	Medications	Comment
7/11 2PM			On maintenance Digitalis leaf 100 mg 8.d. for 6 mos ?PAT ? Parasystolic Tachycardia
6 PM 7:30		E.W 150 PM / 3B 3:30pm / Cardiac Sinus Massage (Quinidine 200mg P.o @ 7:30Pm)	Tō Response
55 7PM		5 minutes later after 14min / Nasal O₂	Spontaneous Conversion to wandering Atrial Pacemaker
30 8PM			Wandering Atrial Pacemaker
7/12 5:30 AM		Midnight Quinidine 200mgm P.o	N.S.R.
30 6PM		@ 6AM Quinidine 200 mg P.o	Sinus rhythm c̄ PAC
		8 PM Digitalis leaf - 100 mgm P.o / Noon - Quinidine 200 mgm P.o	
2 PM			Wandering Atrial Pacemaker
10 PM 3:?M			{? PAT / ? Atrial Fibrillation} ? Parasystolic Tachycardia
15 3PM		Dilantin 250 mg I.v / Dilantin 100mgm I.M	Sinus Rhythm c̄ PAC's
30 4PM	4:15P		
30 4-6PM		Dilantin 250 mgm I.V / 40meg KCl i.v	Tō change in rhythm / Tō " " / Tō " "
6 PM		Nasal O₂ 3 L/min / Cedilanid 0.8 mgm I.v	? Atrial Fibrillation
30 7PM			N.S.R.

The EKG strips appearing above are not exact originals. They have had to be retraced by hand due to difficulties in reproduction of the originals.

PROBLEM LIST

#1. Organic heart disease
   a) probably rheumatic heart disease
   b) generalized cardiac enlargement; MI, AI, AS, ? M.S.
   c) sinus mechanism—atrial fibrillation (now)
   d) congestive heart failure—predominately right-sided
   e) class III consider AV malformation right-sided overload
      —doubt
#2. Goiter with past history of thyrotoxicosis
      Benign vs. toxic—resolved (see PN 5/16/66)
#3. Doubt diabetes mellitus
      Resolved (see PN 5/16/66)
#4. Past history of duodenal ulcer
#5. Azotemia ? etiology (discharge diagnosis—chronic renal
      disease)
      Consider prerenal (doubt with long-standing nature)
      Consider chronic mercurials
#6. R/O-COPE (see PN 5/16/66)

> A flow sheet on a patient such as this, with mul-
> tiple problems, each of which has a long, compli-
> cated history, is an invaluable aid to grasping
> what is essential in the history within a reason-
> able time. It is also necessary to prevent the "pro-
> vincialism in time" that makes the physician
> overinterpret single events, types of therapy,
> and temporary change (e.g., in cardiac rhythm,
> hypertension, and diabetes) which in reality are
> merely ripples on the surface when viewed
> against the twenty-year background of all the
> data. "Off the cuff" oral presentations and pages
> of narrative data are no substitute for a well-
> planned flow sheet in the presentation and com-
> prehension of a complicated case.

DATE	Wgt	V.P. cum	B.P.	Hct.	FBS 24pc	ECG	NA / K	CO₂ / Cl	BUN	PBI / BMR	CHEST FILM	CHOL-ESTEROL	ANTI-THYROID OL	DIGI-TALIS	ORAL THYROID HB+THIO	ORAL QUINI-DINE	REMARKS
Adm #1 12-46	159#	140 / 80				Atrial Fibrillation			14.7		Normal cardiac diameter						Right high saphenous Ligation. Bilateral low Saphena
Adm #2 2-47	145#					Atrial ECG Fibrillation			13.7		cardiac diam hypert A-55 Ca-163		THIO URACIL				Adm. for hyper thyroidism !
3-47	157#					Atrial Fibrillation											placed on digitalis to control rate
4-48	185#					Atrial Fibrillation				+18							Antithyroid MEDS; followed by BMRs
7-50	200#					Atrial Fibrillation											
10-51	190¼#					Atrial ECG Fibrillation											11-51 I-131 262% 4hrs. WNL; DK arrhythmia
1-52						Atrial Fibrillation											
10-54	192					Atrial Fibrillation ECG											10-54: I-131 29% in years. Dk arrhythmia Q
1-55						?A.F. vs? RSR ĉ ECG											4/55 I-131 40 of
Adm #3 2-58	180#			48	1/12	RSR ≤ 1° AV Block	131	100	33	moderate enlargement						Adm. for SOB + edema after of MITRAL stenosis No DX workup
					229	4.8											
4-59						RSR clinically	264										Adm. for ↑ Sx + further DX
11-59						Atrial ECG Fibrillation											
1-27-60						Atrial Fibrillation			7.4								
Adm #4 3-7-60	173#				104.90	Atrial Fibrillation	140 / 5.0	25 / 103	32 / 16	25% ↑ above expected	174					3-10-60 PTT WNL cardiolytics DX: Q MI AF MS
167#										contra parotid disease						I 131 = 4/47 in 48 hrs
Adm #5 3-21-60	160#				73.93	QUINIDINE sinus Arrhythmia			29 to 34 / 1:2			210					
4-14-60	150 / 65					(ventricular Hypertrophy-strain)										Adm for pleurisy"
4-28-60																	

Clinical flow sheet (handwritten, rotated):

DATE	WGT	VP/Venc	B.P.	HCT	FBS 2hr p.p.	ECG	NA+/K+	CO2/Cl	BUN/Creatinine	PBI/BMR	CHEST FILM	TRIAM TERINE/TERINETALIS	DIGITALIS	NAQUA/QUINIDINE	REMARKS
6-61	81 Kg.				108										↑3x← Edema SO
8-62	132#	82.5 K				Atrial tachy cardia with Variable AV block									Naqua begun
11-62	173#	78.5				Sinus arrhyth with rare PVB;									Trace of edema
2-63		77.0 K									"Gross cardio meg"				D/C Naqua; 1+ edema; Naqua resumed
5-63		72.5				Sinus Rhythm c̄ 1° Block. occas. PVC;									Ran out of Quinidine; D/C 4:05 in 4/65
5-65		80.0				RSR (clinical)									
10-65		78.2				Sinus arrhyth c̄ variable A-V Block wandering pacemaker occas PVC;			37 / 2.0		Generalized enlargement. Same as 3-7-63				
3-66	73.1	156					139	43 / 97			No hepatomegaly				
3-66	180#	154	68				138	24	36						Amylase <200
5-10-66	82.0		80					4.6							
5-11-66	179#	26	150 / 90	39.6 / 13.2	90	Atrial fibrill 141		25 / 108	33	4.8	Generalized cardiomegaly c̄ passing in R. Hypers in R.		added KCl↓		hospital admission Rx 250 mgm Na¹ Thorazine Naqua, Naqua c̄ KCl + salt to 1200 mgm
5-23-66	150#	9	140 / 70		171	Atrial fibrill 134		42 / 108	45 / 1.9		Pleural effusion splenic effusion				HOSPITAL DISCHARGE
6-17-66	165#	19	150 / 59			Fibrillation c̄ runs of PVC̄ c̄ Bigeminy	138	41 / 95	35 / 37		① pleural effusion by PEX		D/C		Biventricular failed c̄ OPE tdr m/v
6-21-66	160#	14	160 / 58			Atrial Fibrillation	137	49 / 94	41 / 1.8		= A from 5-23-66				Compensating C#F HOSPITAL ADMISSION
		16						53 / 100	28 / 41						

(Drug-duration columns TRIAM TERINE/TERINETALIS, DIGITALIS, NAQUA, QUINIDINE are shown as shaded bars indicating treatment periods.)

PROBLEM LIST

#1. "Chronic asthma," probably not allergic

#2. Organic heart disease:
   a) hypertensive cardiovascular disease and arteriosclerotic heart disease
   b) atrial fibrillation
   c) cardiomegaly—left ventricular hypertrophy
   d) old inferior wall infarction by EKG

#3. Flatulence, undetermined etiology

#4. Absent pulses, both feet

#5. History of chronic alcoholism

#6. History of alcohol withdrawal (1956) seizures, delerium tremens

#7. Hepatomegaly—"delete" 4/15/66

#8. History of lues

#9. Post transurethral resection in 1962

DATE	BP	$\dot{p}$	EKG	Hct	Wt.	Na+/K+	Cl-/CO2	BUN/Cr.	QUINIDINE	RESERPINE	NAQUA	DIGITALIS	KCL	H.O.
6/54														
4/57	160/120				193									V.2·91-46
5/58	210/130				213									
5/62	130/120		SINUS TACH		209					0.75				LVH + Strain on EKG. Cardiomegaly on chest film
7/62	240/120		2:1 BLOCK	44		141/4.5	100/13.5	11/1			6	100		EKG: 1° AV Block, 2:1 block, + occ. PVC – Dig. toxicity?
8/62	170/90				195									
10/63	180/140	80												Marked cardiomegaly Bilat. pleural effusion
11/63	180/130	100	1° BLOCK											
12/63	170/110	90												
4/64	230/130				187									
6/64	190/110	72			185									
8/64	190/110				187				10					
2/65	190/120	80							20		4	100		
1/66	180/90	82	ATRIAL FIB.		183	145/3.8	95	10/1						
4/66	190/110	100-115												EKG: Freq. PVCs & PAC. prob. dig. toxicity.

1966 DATE	BP	P	EKG	Hct.	Wt.	Na+/K+	Cl/CO₂	BUN/CR	QUINIDINE	QUINAGLUTE	RESERPINE	DIGITALIS	KCl	HYDRODIURIL	H.O.
4/12/66	150/105	80	ATR. FIB.	41	170	$\frac{146}{3.7}$	$\frac{100}{37}$	21/		20	4	100			
4/13-	140/110				178										↓: 2-9-46
4/16	120/90	75			177										
4/19	140/110	70	NSR.		171										CARDIOVERSION - 4/21
4/22	140/90	84													DISCHARGE
4/28	150/90	84	2° BL. PVCs.		174										OPC
5/5	150/90	84			174										OPC
5/20	150/96	65													CGH ADMISSION
5/23			NSR.		173										
6/2	148/84	80	VAR. Block												DISCHARGE
6/5	170/110	76	Toxic	44						90					
6/29	120/70	68			180.4							300			CGH ADM. - ? DIG. Toxicity
7/8	140/102	96			181.5							$\frac{100}{qid}$			CONG. FAILURE
7/12	150/100	88	1° BL. PVC.		182.6										EW VISIT - S.O.B. EDEMA; GIVEN HERE 1.0 cc. IM.

1966 DATE	BP	P	EKG	Hct.	Wt.	Na+/K+	Cl-/CO2	BUN/CR.	QUINIDINE	QUINETH.	RESERPINE	MAGLIA	DIGITALIS	MERC.	HYDRA-LAZINE	H.O. U.J. 91-46
7/15	130/80	72			183.6 / 212 K				20 Q6H	40			100 QID	1cc	200	
7/30	156/102	67			81.8											
8/12	190/120	102			81.2					40						
8/16	200/110	100			81.6									1cc		EW-DYSPNEA
8/26	100/110	96			83											
8/30					83.2					70				1cc		EW. S.O.B, orthopnea,
9/5	160/110	116			82.5											
9/21	160/106					130/3.1	:34	13/-								CONTINUED DYSPNEA, ORTHOPNEA, PALPITATIONS
10/3	120/?				77.2											CHGH-? DIG. TOXICITY
10/6	170/110	75			77.2											
10/7	170/115	80			78.6											
10/10	140/90	75			79.5	140/5.3	103/31	18/4.0						1cc		2gm. NACL
10/11	170/130	95			75.9											
10/18					80 (clothes)							10/14				0.5 NaCl 2gm. Nacl

PROBLEM LIST

#1. Right-upper-lobe abscess

#2. Bronchogenic carcinoma with metastases

#3. Weight loss and dysphagia, secondary to #2

#4. Malnutrition and anemia

#5. Abnormal voice

#6. Chronic alcoholism

#7. External hemorrhoid

> This flow sheet reveals at a glance the time relationships among the cultures, the antibiotics, and the temperatures; among the serum iron (should there be an iron binding capacity), the drugs, and the weight gain. One immediately sees when the bronchoscopy occurred in the course. One might raise the question: What was the goal as far as the hematocrit was concerned?

DATE	WT lbs.	Hct.	Rec'k Temp	SPUTUM CULTURE (ALSO BLOOD)	MEDS IV	Na	K	Cl	CO₂	BUN	Cr	C.C.R.	
2/28	89	23	39	NON GRP A β STREP	PEN	126	3.9	92	24	10		Sx:	
3/1		21 (2 units blood)	38⁸	PNEUMO STAPH AUREUS (PEN+RES) HELM (PARA GLCU ETC-)	12 m.u.	33		25.5		1.0			SERUM Fe: 20
2	27	27	39⁶	STAPH (PEN+RES) AERO BACTER ALPHA STREP	6 m.u.							Doing Well	
3			39⁴	KLEBSIELLA TYPE 4								Doing well	
4		28	39¹	STAPH AUREUS								Doing well	
5			38⁸									Doing well	
6	95		38⁶		KANA CHLOROMYCIN	129	3.0	90	31.5	10	1.0	Doing well	
7		27	39¹									Doing Well	PO KCl
8			38⁸									Doing well	˙ᵎ SERUM FE: 47
9	97½		40									Doing well	
10			38¹			130	4.4	97	21.5	9		˙˙	˙˙
11			39⁴									˙˙	˙˙
12			38²									˙˙	˙˙
13			40²									˙˙	˙˙
14													

← BRONCHOSCOPY

← BRONCHOSCOPY

PROBLEM LIST

#1. Laennec's cirrhosis with hepatic failure

#2. Acute renal failure

#3. Gastrointestinal bleeding

#4. Staphylococcus enteritis

#5. Deceased

This flow sheet illustrates the value of having all the parameters immediately available in order to make quick and reliable decisions concerning volume, free water (tonicity), potassium, and acid-base. On August 6, for example, the volume parameters show an increase in venous pressure, no fall in weight, no dramatic change in hematocrit, and yet a marked fall in blood pressure. What was done to evaluate cardiac output? It will be noted that the free-water decisions may have led to a serum sodium of 119, whereas the patient was admitted with one of 138. Exactly why and how much free water was given? It will be noted that the potassium reached 6.6 before KCl was discontinued. Why was therapy handled in this way? Why is the calorie column so empty before August 1? What should be the management of the blood urea nitrogen in the face of all these difficulties? It is from data such as this, observed over and over again, that students slowly absorb the significant factors in managing difficult problems.

In such cases it should be pointed out to the student that one can rarely predict with confidence the course of any given parameter. Any

INPUT — OUTPUT

Date	B.P.	P.R.	Wgt (LBS)	CVP mmH2O	HCT	Na/K Cl/CO2 BUN/pH creat.	Calories Daily	Cumulative	Input Daily	Cumulative	Output Daily	Cumulative	Stools	Remarks — E. W.
7/24					34	135 2.4/.25								
7/26			150			136/2.5 97/28					20/			Remarks
7/27			150½			130/3.4 93/27.5	140	1410	700	700	28/			SAR estimate 7/27 was
7/28						136/5.3 100/35.0	3085	5500	1700	3600	29/			Patient 5% dehydrated
7/29			841			135/3.9 103/33.5	3600	9100	250	2850	40/			
7/30			151			152/3.3 99/35	2500	11600	925					
7/31							2570	14170	900	4675				Paracentesis for distention (Relief) → guess ~ 2 Liters Via L. Eckage ≈ 250cc aspirated
8/1	140/70	90				125/2.6 100/11.5	4380	18550	1400	6100	57/		800 →	NGT placed in stomach to Relieve gastric distension ~ 900cc gastric ~ material Removed
8/2	120/70	110				129/2.5 21	2300	20800	3000	9100	68/5.9			KCl D/C (oral) 1000 cc urine out
8/3	100/60	96	151	40mm	31	/3.8 67 7/18	2700	23600	400	9500	67			24 hr. urine 15 mag NR : 27 Mg K + 25 gm Gilbumin given in 20 minutes
8/4			154	30-40	29	118/4.3 87/31.5	900	24500	110	9600	69/6.4		6 Loose stools	Many Tubular casts seen in spun Tubular sediment Dx made 2 Ranment Staphlococci
8/5	70/40		151¾	30-40	30	120/4.0 20	2600	27100	200	9900			5 Loose	Blood - 1 unit BP between 7/40 – 70/40 all day 2 bounding pulse
8/6	60/60 70/40		153	110 to 140		125/3.6 93/20	3310	30000	300	10200	7½/6		No stool Recent	Begin maintenance 2 Boli Electrolyte solution Liponal Begun
8/7	82/40		—	122/134		17½/5.4 17	1220	31.2	350	10.5	81/		No stool Recent	Maintenance Fluids plus Liponal + Plodox
8/8	90/50		147¾			124/5.1 140/11.3	1110	32.3	100	10.6	77/		4 Loose stools	Maintenance Fluids plus Liponal + Glodvox Plus
8/9	80/60				29	131/5.2 140 25 37	1000	33.3	100	10.7	94/		Semi formed	
8/10														Levophed in C? mgm/500 cc Run at 0.3c mgm/min ↓ BP

teacher or older physician who makes such statements as "the patient should have had three liters of fluid last night with that rising blood urea nitrogen," or "That dose of digitalis (or that injection of that amount of calcium) is absolutely wrong," or "That patient obviously has classical ——, and there is no question about exactly what she needs," is a clinician whose experience has not included the detailed analysis and following up of the data on multiple, interacting problems. Although one might have recognized the possibility of hyponatremia in the face of a given water load in the above case, one could not be assured of such a response. There are in complex cases so many forces operating which we do not fully understand, and so many forces unperceived and yet to be detected, that our whole system of management must be based on the assumption (and awareness) of possible error in all decisions coupled with data systems designed for "feedback" and corrective action. Flow sheets and titled progress notes are the most crucial portion of an effective feedback loop in medical care.

7

THE DISCHARGE SUMMARY

The discharge summary should be problem-oriented. Only that historical, physical, and laboratory information necessary to the future analysis or management of a problem should be included. For example, a pneumococcal pneumonia that has been diagnosed and treated successfully requires very little notice in the summary, whereas abdominal pain that was never completely understood or resolved should be described at length so that the next physician, in his office or in an emergency room, will receive as much help as possible as he grapples with this recurring and poorly understood problem.

The need for and structure of discharge summaries will vary greatly with the situation. Ultimately, with a computerized record providing all the data on a given problem in sequence at any point in time, discharge summaries may not even be necessary. At the other extreme is the state of information that may be expected when a patient with many difficult problems has been followed for years and several thick volumes of old records of the traditional type—a trial to all those who encounter them—have accumulated. In the latter situation it is sometimes convenient to write an over-all, problem-oriented summary and an accompanying flow sheet to help clarify the many tangled and confusing events. The following discharge summary was written on such a complicated case. It was accompanied by a flow sheet, which has been omitted here, as have the summaries of the problems between #1 and #22.

EXAMPLE OF DISCHARGE SUMMARY

This was the 4th —— Hospital admission for this 27-year-old, married, white man with multiple problems.

Problem #1. Rheumatoid arthritis, atypical

SYMPTOMATIC. This is the patient's principal disease. The onset of this disease was November 7, 1963; at this time he developed periodic chills, fever, muscle and joint pains. Fever and chills persisted, and he was admitted to the hospital for the first time in November, 1963. Diagnosis at that time was acute rheumatic fever. Since that time he has had a course unique in its variability. Predominant symptoms were polymyalgia, pain in the joints, principally those of the upper extremity, and intermittent fevers. Many diagnoses were entertained during the initial 3 years of the patient's illness, and included rheumatoid arthritis, periarteritis nodosa, and rheumatic fever.

He first presented to this hospital approximately 4 years prior to admission when he presented to the Outpatient Department several weeks after discharge from his first hospitalization at —— Hospital. His complaints at that time were migratory polyarthritis and a sore throat of 1.5-months duration. He was then followed at other hospitals, until he again came to the Outpatient Clinic about 15 months prior to admission. At this time he complained of pain in his right thorax, and of transient temperature spikes to 40°. He also had a perirectal abscess at this time. Symptomatically, a remission of sorts was achieved between 12 and 4 months prior to this admission; during this time, the pain in his hands, wrists, and shoulders was less, he was able to ambulate and even to work although still troubled occasionally by muscle aches and fever.

The present admission was prompted by persistent pain in his joints and muscles, spiking fevers, and acutely by vomiting. His hospital course has been one of very gradual but inexorable deterioration. "Remissions," or periods when joint symptoms and muscle pains were controllable by the patient with his usual dose of analgesics, were punctuated by acute flares of his disease which now is called rheumatoid arthritis but felt to be an atypical form of same. The flares are accompanied by autonomic lability, including fever, tachycardia, and hypotension; this may well represent transient adrenal insufficiency at times of stress.

The two involved families in this case, that is, the patient's mother and sister, and his wife and children, all show great concern for his welfare, sometimes to the extent that friction arises between the two family groups. His disease has caused significant adjustments in both financial and social life of both these family groups. At present there remain large medical bills outstanding and doubtless the friction between the two family groups arises in part from this and in part from lack of effective communication. At present he is somewhat depressed at the prospect of leaving the place where he has spent the past 4 months; he is being given reinforcement here and will no doubt be able to adjust satisfactorily to his new environment.

OBJECTIVE: Objective data in favor of the diagnosis of rheumatoid arthritis are few—multiple latex fixation tests for rheumatoid arthritis have been negative but on several occasions have been positive at dilutions as high as 1:80. Biopsy of a nodule in the occipital area approximately 2 months prior to discharge was characteristic of a rheumatoid nodule. Arthritis consultants have felt that the course of the disease, with some response to steroids, is also characteristic of rheumatoid arthritis. Other diagnostic procedures have included multiple estimations of LE factor which have all been negative; antinuclear factors which have all been negative; muscle biopsy on one occasion was normal, and on another showed slight denervation atrophy of one muscle; and electromyogram was also characteristic of denervation. Antibodies to thyroid were not discovered. Febrile and cold agglutinins were negative, but an increased complement level was determined on one occasion. A renal biopsy 4 months prior to discharge showed membranous glomerulonephritis, with interstitial infiltration, possibly pyelonephritic in nature.

Physical examination reveals a chronically ill white man with blood pressure 170/90. Other positive physical findings related to the rheumatoid arthritis are: palpable liver and spleen, swollen and tender joints, greater in the upper extremities than in the lower, and greater distally than proximally. The patient is in pain almost constantly and requires narcotics as detailed below for control.

therapeutic: Therapy has consisted of

(1) Steroids. The patient was treated initially at hospitals in Georgia, Tennessee, West Virginia, and at —— Hospital in Cleveland with various steroid preparations, leading to some relief. He was treated by this hospital initially with Prednisone, at a dose of 60 to 80 mg. per day. At the beginning of this hospitalization he was also begun on hydrocortisone; the dose was soon increased to 240 mg. per day. This dose was maintained until approximately 1.5 months prior to discharge when a gradual decreasing regimen was begun; his present dose is 160 mg./day in 4 divided doses. It is felt that continued very gradual reduction should be attempted. Throughout his course here, he has required parenteral hydrocortisone in the management of his acute flares; doses used have been 50 to 100 mg. intravenously or intramuscularly every 4 to 6 hours.

(2) Analgesics. During the initial part of his disease, the patient was managed with many nonnarcotic analgesics, including Demerol, Darvon, and large doses of aspirin. It is also known that he was addicted to and withdrawn from morphine during his past course. During this hospitalization he has been maintained on methadone, 7.5 to 10 mg. intramuscularly every 4 hours. There has been no evidence of intolerance, although he is certainly addicted to this drug (see diagnosis #23).

· · · · · ·

Problem #22. Persistent Elevation of Antistreptolys in O Titer

SYMPTOMATIC: See diagnosis #1; sore throat was a prominent part of the beginning of this man's illness.

OBJECTIVE: Multiple determinations of the ASO titer have ranged from 500 to 833 Todd units. Group A beta streptococci have been isolated from this patient (see diagnosis #14).

THERAPEUTIC: One week prior to discharge, the patient was begun on tetracycline, 1 gm./day; we feel that this should be continued for at least a month in an attempt to eradicate both active streptococci and possibly present L-forms from him. Whether or not this has any bearing on his basic disease is pure conjecture.

Problem #23. Methadone Addiction

SYMPTOMATIC: The patient is rarely able to miss one of his scheduled doses of this analgesic. Withdrawal symptoms occurred when given a narcotic antagonist approximately 2 months prior to admission.

Problem #24. Penicillin Allergy

This is based on a transient rash which appeared on the patient's nose during penicillin therapy 5 years prior to admission. He has not been given penicillin since; there is no history of anaphylactic or urticarial reaction.

CONDITION ON DISCHARGE: Poor

PROGNOSIS: Poor

DURATION OF DISABILITY: Lifelong

RECOMMENDATIONS: 1. Discharge to —— for extended care.

2. Return February 21 to Arthritis and Eye Clinics.

3. Medications:* 1. Colace 100 mg po bid

2. Allopurinol 100 mg po q8h

3. Folic acid 5 mg po qd

4. Elixir potassium chloride 25 cc (mEq) po qid 2000 cc

5. Digoxin 0.25 mg po qd

6. Maalox 30 cc po q2h while awake 1 cc

7. Pyridoxine 50 mg po bid

8. Robitussin 5 cc po q6h times 5 days

9. Tetracycline 250 mg po qid for 21 days

10. Hydrocortisone 40 mg po q6h

11. Methadone 7.5 mg IM q4h prn

12. IPPB with 4:1 Aerolone for 15 minutes tid times 5 days

---

* Abbreviations:
bid = twice daily
IPPB = intermittent positive pressure breathing
mEq = mille equivalents
po = by mouth

prn = as necessary
qd = each day
q2h, etc. = every 2 hours, etc.
qid = 4 per day

8

A CASE HISTORY

The following medical record of a 79-year-old patient with multiple problems is taken at random from the files of two physicians currently conducting a busy general practice in a small town in Maine. Their internship training nine years ago was based upon problem-oriented patient records and care. One may not necessarily agree with their medical decisions, but the manner in which each problem is formulated, pursued, and related to the other problems makes it possible for the reader to assess quality of medical care in terms of the physician's thoroughness and analytical capacity.

There have been minor, but useful, modifications in form since the time of the rotating internship of these practitioners. In the initial plan, not only the number but also the title of each problem is now used, facilitating even more rapid audit of the physician's approach to a particular situation. It will also be noted that problems #8, hiatus hernia, and #9, diverticulosis, were not listed at the time of admission even though they were known. Instead, the physician entered them in the "master" problem list, on the face of the record, when they seemed to become relevant. This procedure is not recommended. Rather, all significant problems should be entered as soon as they are known, including those that are inactive or resolved. Also, progress notes should follow a form similar to that described earlier, in which the physician first discusses the problem from the patient's point of view (subjectively, *Sx*), then states all appropriate objective data (*Obj*) pertinent to the patient's problem, states current treatment (*Rx*), gives any new interpretations (*Imp*) and, finally (*Plan*) discusses the plan for the next interval. Other minor anomalies may be observed.

MEDICAL RECORD FROM A GENERAL PRACTICE*

Problem List ["Master" List, on the Face of the Record]

#1. Rheumatoid arthritis

#2. Anemia

#3. Neuritis

#4. Edema

#5. Depression—personality change

#6. Fever of unknown origin (see note 5/11)

#7. Vomiting (see note 5/18)

#8. Hiatus hernia

#9. Diverticulosis

#10. Pneumonia (see note 6/4)

#11. Gall bladder disease (see note 6/6)

#1. RHEUMATOID ARTHRITIS. Beginning about 1963 the patient [aged 79] began having multiple joint symptoms characterized by pain and some limitation of motion. She has been followed by Dr. —— for this since that time. She had a positive latex fixation test at that time, a uric acid of 2.0. In 1966 the knees were injected with Aristocort with symptomatic relief. She has continued to have a

---

*The following abbreviations are used in this record:

ABD = abdominal	G.I. = gastrointestinal
AG = albumin/globulin	hct = hematocrit
BP = blood pressure	hgb = hemoglobin
BUN = blood urea nitrogen	HPI = hospital present illness
cal = calorie	HS = at bedtime
cath = catheter	IM = intramuscular
DTR = deep tendon reflexes	LA = left arm
E.N.T. = ear, nose, and throat	mem = membrane

moderate amount of joint symptoms although no severe deformity of any joint.

Therapy has consisted of salicylates which she continues to take. 15 grains every four hours, prednisone being started in September 1966, with dramatic improvement for about a month, but persistent symptoms since that brief improvement, her regular daily dose being 5 milligrams twice a day although at times at home she has taken 20 to 25 milligrams per day. Additionally she took aralen temporarily without significant improvement.

#2. ANEMIA. In February 1966 the patient was found to have a hematocrit of 29 to 31% marked-hypochromia, multiple stools positive for occult blood, hiatus hernia demonstrated by X ray, diverticulosis of the colon and negative sigmoidoscopy. A folic acid was 2 (normal is 5 to 6). Serum albumin 3.0, globulin 3.0. No PBI, serum iron or reticulocyte count or bone marrow were done. A serum B-12 level was normal. In December 1966 hematocrit was 26%, bilirubin less than 1, and in March 1967 hematocrit was 39%. Treatment has consisted of multiple vitamins, temporarily on En-Cebrin F but currently on a simple multiple vitamin and thiamine intramuscularly daily. No folic acid. Additionally she has had several blood transfusions and had received iron in the past although is not on iron. The hematocrit today is reported at 27–28% with a normal white count and differential.

#3. NEURITIS. For approximately two months the patient has had considerable paresthesias particularly in her feet, described as

mic = microscopic	B/P = blood pressure
neuro = neurological	prot = protein
nl = normal	q3 = every three
NG = naso-gastric	q.4.h. = every four hours
NSR = normal sinus rhythm	R = respirations
ō = without	R/O = rule out
P = pulse	spec = special
P&R = pelvic and rectal	T = temperature
PBI = protein bound iodine	U.T.I. = urinary tract infection
PC = after meals	WBC = white blood count
P.O. = by mouth	

painful sensations with numbness even at rest. Dr. —— found absent reflexes in the lower extremities and absent vibratory sense. Pain was intact. Peripheral pulses were normal. She has had marked peripheral edema the past two or three months. The cause of this neuritis has remained obscure.

#4. EDEMA. Marked peripheral edema and facial edema has been noted for several months. The last serum albumin reported was in February 1966–3.0. A 2-hour PC blood sugar was 150 milligrams percent in December 1966 and potassium of 5.3. BUN 20 milligrams percent and negative urinalysis on 3/67. Chest X ray at that time revealed slight cardiac enlargement. This was a portable film, but was not particularly suggestive of congestive failure. Blood pressures have been in the normal range of 150/80, a grade II murmur has been present. She has not been digitalized. She has been on salt restriction because of her steroids and has received Diuril in the past without significant effect on the edema.

#5. DEPRESSION—PERSONALITY CHANGE. The patient relates that she has not felt well for a number of years, seeming to date this most closely to the death of Mrs. ——, the lady for whom she worked some eight or ten years following her husband's death. She had a very close relationship with this lady, was very fond of her and often thinks of her now. She feels she began having her joint pains at about the time of her death and has never worked since that time. She does not believe there has been any impairment in her thinking or memory. She does believe there has been some voice change in the form of hoarseness or lowering and slight temperature intolerance to cold. She finds herself crying a lot. Recently in the home the nurses have noted that she is temporarily disoriented and is hallucinating images such as animals. At times she is not very communicative, at other times seems somewhat hostile, fearful that anyone will touch her and this will be painful. A recent trial on Elavil was without any apparent benefit. She is currently on Thorazine 25 milligrams every four hours with little objective or symptomatic improvement and she is complaining of a dry, sore tongue, possibly related to this.

Review of Systems

Central Nervous System: Denies headaches or dizziness.

Special senses: Vision seems fair, although seems to fluctuate; is able to read the paper and hears fairly well.

Respiratory: Infrequent colds. Denies pneumonia or chronic cough. Sleeps on one pillow.

Cardiovascular: No known heart trouble other than slight cardiac enlargement by X ray. Grade II systolic murmur noted in the past. Blood pressures have been 150/80. Peripheral pulses have been intact in spite of the marked peripheral edema and facial edema.

Gastrointestinal: Hiatus hernia by X ray in 1966. Denies indigestion however. Also diverticulosis by X ray. The patient has not been on any ulcer prophylactic regime. Occult blood in stool has been noted on at least two admissions.

Genitourinary: No known kidney trouble. About 1 x nocturia. BUN's of 18 and 20 milligrams percent on previous admissions with negative urinalysis. This also repeated today.

Musculo Skeletal: See HPI no. 1

Hematologic: See HPI no. 2

Metabolic: Potassium of 3.8 in December 1966. Weight is said to be fairly stable at about 145 to 155.

Physical Examination

B/P 150/80 LA. Pulse 96 and regular. T—100. Weight.
This is an elderly lady who has a low-pitched, froggy-type voice, however the Thorazine may very well be contributing significantly to this. There is rather marked puffiness of her face, eyelids. Her affect is rather flat, yet her memory seems good although her recall seems slow. Physical examination completed in usual manner.

Problem List

#1 *Rheumatoid arthritis*—maintained on aspirin gram 15 q.4.h. and prednisone 5 milligrams twice a day.

#2 *Anemia*—probably related to blood loss by G.I. tract but also rule out persistent folic acid deficiency and hypothyroidism. R/O myxedema & folic acid deficiency.

#3   *Peripheral neuritis*—uncertain etiology.

#4   *Peripheral edema*—uncertain etiology—malnutrition.

#5   *Depression and memory impairment or slowing up of thought processes*—uncertain etiology—myxedema.

Plans

#1   Continue same regime although would suggest elevating head of bed, addition of belladonna and Maalox PC and HS.

#2* Serum iron, folic acid, total protein AG ratio. PBI.

#3   Continue multiple vitamin possibly should add folic acid. Folic acid level to be checked.

#4   Evaluate serum protein level as well as PBI.

#5   Probably I am overly impressed by her skin texture suggesting myxedema and her voice changes which may be due to the Thorazine. If the PBI is normal, then perhaps a more vigorous or intensive trial on antidepressants, more rapidly acting such as Pertofrane or Aventyl should be given or possibly shock therapy employed.

[Progress Note] 5/11

#1   *R.A.*—No change—unable to take meds today.

#2   *Anemia*—Serum Fe 36. Folic acid NL. Hgb. 8.5 gms today.

#3   *Neuritis*—No change.

#4   *Edema*—No change clinically—PBI + Total I normal.
      (Severe hypo-albuminemia.)
      Cal. count + 1 spec. prot. intake per day.
      Plan was to pass N. G. tube if Dr. —— (E.N.T.) found no lesion and he did not on exam today—force feed via tube for a few weeks.

---

* Note how readily one detects the absence of stool guaiacs in these initial plans for this particular problem. The physician did recognize this aspect in the discussion above, also in a later numbered and titled progress note in which three negative stools are discussed.

#5 *Depression*—Patient agitated during nite—lost weight—given Thorazine 25 mgm @ midnite (had 75 mgm Elavil yesterday) today semiresponsive, unable to take orally and has *low grade fever.**

Physical Examination

B.P. 140/70. P—80 & reg. T—101ᴿ. R—32/min.
Responds to voice occasionally—pain regularly—not intelligible speech.
EENT—Nl. except dry mucous mem.
NECK—Supple—carotids nl.
LUNGS—clear, aerate well.
HEART—NSR—Grade II sys. murmur—ō gallop, rub, etc.
ABD.—Soft, obese—? RLQ tenderness & ? RLQ mass.
P&R—Deferred.
NEURO—responds as noted—DTR's symmetrical, depressed ō pathologic reflexes.
SKIN—Several ecchymotic areas & superficial abrasions, marked generalized edema—waxy turgor to skin.
CHEST X RAY—Cardiomegaly
WBC—10,000+
URINE—Not obtained.
IMP.—Same plus—#6 fever of unknown origin**
PLAN—Admit for observation.

[Progress Note] 5/13

#2 *Anemia*—will recheck hgb. hct. today—to get IM Fe—20 cc Imferon.

---

* The pattern of the physician's thought is suggested as he discusses the semi-responsiveness under the depression, momentarily couples the fever with both, and then quickly decides to follow the fever as a separate problem under #6 after finding a supple neck and no localizing signs. Should he have done a lumbar puncture before he decided to leave the semiresponsiveness with the depression and drugs and formulate the fever as a separate problem? A problem list and titled progress notes reveal the context in which thoughts occur and actions are taken. Knowledge of content without context can be useless or even misleading.
** See note above.

#4 Edema—malnutrition—#16 plastic tube inserted yesterday.

#5 Depression—perhaps a little more responsive. Wants water P.O. —off psychotropic drugs.

#6 Fever of unknown origin—will insert Foley cath. to preserve skin; and evaluate U.T.I.; 540 cc; Mic—neg.

[Progress Note] 5/15

#4 Edema—nutrition—tolerating NG feeding.
750 cal—150 a q 3—will increase to 350 a q 3—1,000 cal/24°.

The record continues for another six months, with gradual evolution of all the problems and remarkable resolution of some, such as the edema, the poor nutrition, and the psychiatric difficulties. Problem-oriented discharge summaries similar to the example presented in Chapter 7, do much to facilitate rapid assessment of cases such as this.

9

IMPLICATIONS OF THE PROBLEM-ORIENTED RECORD

The structured, problem-oriented medical record provides a focus for constructive action in ameliorating a variety of difficulties now besetting medicine: medical problems dealt with out of context; inefficiency in practice (as evidenced by the excessively strenuous burdens upon most physicians and the differences in the quality and amount of care received by inpatients and outpatients); lack of continuity of care; the apparent inapplicability of "basic science" facts and principles; inefficiency in education (resulting from improvised and undisciplined rounds and conferences); and finally, the absence of meaningful audit in the practice of medicine.

PROBLEMS OUT OF CONTEXT

Multiple problems may interact, and sophisticated understanding and management of any one of them requires at least an awareness of all of them. Where the findings, for instance, show heart failure and azotemia, it is apparent that the right treatment for one may be the wrong treatment for the other, and the need for skillful management is obvious. In other situations the interaction may not be so obvious—as in paroxysmal hypertension, dehydration, and hypovolemia. In such cases physicians always risk faulty interpretation by treating problems out of context.

For example, in the list of problems in Fig. 5 (Chapter 3), the management of dehydration in problem #3 dramatically improved problem #1, accelerated hypertension. The volume indicators and other appropriate variables were followed, using a flow sheet, as intravenous volume expanders were given. Aggressive conventional drug therapy of the marked diastolic hypertension, employed out of context, could have had serious consequences.

The interdependence of social and medical problems is immediately revealed by a complete list of problems. An awareness of a social problem—lack of proper heating in the house, for instance—is more fundamental to the management of a medical problem such as pneumonia than the management of other associated medical problems—arthritis or a urinary tract infection. Common-sense approaches to total care are facilitated by a complete problem list. The medical literature is replete with papers on single entities from series of patients (for example, myocardial infarction, cancer of the colon, or pneumonia) in which no complete problem list for each patient was systematically presented. A paper may talk about X per cent mortality for perforated ulcer when, for example, what it should really be saying is Y per cent if heart failure is also on the list or Z per cent if another problem or no others are present. Pneumococcal pneumonia alone may well be a different disease from pneumococcal pneumonia in the presence of azotemia. Potent drugs are administered, and major management decisions made for specific problems taken out of context. It is no wonder that controversies in medicine abound; the present lack of technique for the recording and presentation of data on multiple problems almost guarantees chaos.

Until well-conceived problem lists are the rule rather than the exception, so that the problems of most patients are dealt with in scrupulous context, the fragmentation of care in today's specialty clinics and wards, and the fragmentation of the survey of that care on rounds and in conferences, can never be attacked seriously. The physician must learn how to move easily from a single-minded focus on one problem to attention to the total list and the interrelations of many problems, much as a biochemist meticulously purifies and studies an enzyme in a scheme of reactions and then returns to consider its relation to the others. He does not, and could not, get basic data on all the enzymes simultaneously in the interest of total biochemistry—or the "art of biochemistry"—nor does he work on only one and arbitrarily dismiss the others as of little concern. The essential combination of the clarification of single problems and the integration of multiple problems is greatly facilitated by a medical record that is structured upon a total problem list and titled progress notes. Since the human body is a complex group of systems, each of which can develop abnormalities that reverberate through the other systems to varying degrees, the specialist, as a responsible scientist, must know the variables in the total system as they affect his specialized judgment and action. A patient's intuitive demand for a "whole doctor" is completely consistent with the demands that good science and a sense of all the relevant factors in any patient's illness impose upon the specialist, quite apart from general considerations of the need for "primary" physicians, total care, and humanitarianism.

The fragmentation of single diagnostic entities that results from listing individual but related findings separately is not a legitimate complaint against a complete list of problems. If a complete analysis is done on each finding, integration of related findings occurs with clarity and inevitability. Failure to integrate findings into a valid single entity can almost always be traced to incomplete understanding of all the implications of one or all of them. If a beginner enters cardiomegaly, edema, hepatomegaly, and shortness of breath as four separate problems, he thereby emphatically admits that he does not recognize cardiac failure when he sees it. But the important point is that nothing is lost. On the contrary, the interest of more experienced observers is immediately aroused, the patient's problems are

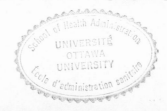

combined as appropriate under a single heading on the original list, and they are carried one step closer to diagnosis and treatment. The system does not prevent analysis and integration; it merely reveals the extent to which they are performed and defines the level of sophistication at which the physician functions.

THE BURDENS UPON THE PHYSICIAN

A scientist prefers to choose his own problems, to determine a sequence of action, and then to spend as much time as necessary in solving the problems. A physician does not choose his problems; they are chosen for him by the patient, who also initiates the problem-solving encounter.

Many symptomatic problems demanding immediate care might have received organized attention and at the physician's initiative in a less acute phase, if, instead of being ignored by the too-busy doctor (who was dashing off random notes on the acute episode of some other previously neglected situation), they had been identified in that phase and followed systematically in numbered, titled progress notes. A physician should always examine deliberately the patient's complete problem list. If his time is limited, he should establish priorities and direct attention to those problems having the greatest potential for moving into the acute phase. The rule should be: *When the physician is under pressure, he should do what he does very well; he should select the problem or problems for immediate action, and he should never attempt to deal with all the problems superficially for the mere sake of having dealt with them.* If this approach is followed, the work reflected in each titled progress note can become a precisely defined building block, all effort can be cumulative, and sharply increased efficiency can result. Lack of time is not a legitimate argument against keeping data in order. Form leads to ultimate economy of time in almost all human endeavors.

When records such as those presented in the last chapter can be kept by busy practitioners, the excuse of lack of time cannot be regarded as tenable. Medical students and physicians can be taught to deal with heavy work loads, to set priorities, and to direct paramedical help wisely. The medical record is an ideal instrument for achieving these educational goals. We should not assess a physician's effectiveness by the amount of time he spends with patients or the sophistication of his specialized techniques. Rather we should judge him on the *completeness and accuracy of the data base he creates as he starts his work, the speed and economy with which he obtains patient data, the adequacy of his formulation of all the problems, the intelligence he demonstrates as he carefully treats and follows each problem, and the total quantity of acceptable care he is able to deliver.*

INPATIENT CARE VS. OUTPATIENT CARE

There is, of course, much in the organization of medicine in the medical schools and the community that militates against efficiency in administering effective, acceptable care to the community as a whole. Medical institutions and some practicing physicians have never been formally assigned a specific population for whose health they are responsible. Were such assignments made, more attention could be directed to the prevention of disease and to the care and education of the ambulatory patient. If a patient is assigned to a physician when the patient is asymptomatic, the appearance or progression of serious but preventable problems is a measure of the physician's failure. As matters now stand, if the patient sees the physician in late-stage disease, then the physician is likely to be praised for the solution or alleviation of problems that should have been prevented in the first place.

The training years of a physician are inpatient oriented and so by definition emphasize late-stage disease. A patient in the outpatient clinics of many training institutions has available to him the merest fraction of the physician time that would have been available to him as an inpatient. He gets even less time, proportionately, from the nurse, the dietitian, and the laboratory technician. Indeed, on the basis of a few moments of hasty advice he goes home from the clinic to be his own laboratory technician, his own nurse, his own pharmacist, and his own dietitian. When problems are in the subtle early stages (e.g., a confusing case of angina, early kidney disease, or eclampsia—or the faint beginnings of appendicitis in an older person with multiple problems), the patient may receive five minutes of time from an inexperienced and unsophisticated physician in the clinic or the accident room. If a misjudgment is made, the patient goes home to struggle with the consequences himself. There is no reinforcement by nurses, residents, and older physicians, who normally would monitor and adjust therapy continuously in the hospital as new evidence was accumulated. On the other hand, when the patient's disease is a massive myocardial infarct, overwhelming and obvious pyelitis and septicemia, or a perforated appendix, he is taken to wards where, during hours, days, and weeks of rounds and conferences by full professors, residents, and consultants, the now obvious diagnosis is confirmed, treatment is followed up, and the metabolic and anatomic complexity and chaos that are the inevitable result of long-neglected multiple problems are meticulously dissected. The practical consequences are that academic excitement and intellectual stimulation are harvested from delayed maintenance. Many such problems could have been foreseen and prevented by a system that emphasized better care and more patient education in the clinics, the accident rooms, and the community. This is a subtle and demanding aim, worthy of the best minds available in medical education. I do not say that students and house officers should not learn the sophisticated and complicated maneuvers of inpatient medicine for very sick people, but I do mean to say that inefficient and nonproductive discussions among inpatient physicians in the name of sophistication and scholarship cannot be allowed to take place at the expense of responsibilities in ambulatory care.

Every medical student and house officer should be assigned a population of patients, both ambulatory and bedridden; he should have a complete data base and list of problems on each, and he should be taught priorities, assigning first priority to those problems that are reversible in people who still have their lives to live, their families to support, and their contributions to make to society. A student must be taught economy of action and thought in the ward and must be directed to emphasize his responsibilities in the clinic, so that people will not be obliged to become very sick before they get his attention. He should stay up as late in a record room getting ready for a clinic patient as he does in a ward treating terminal patients in shock. Faculties must reverse the time-ratio of ward to clinic medicine and put to an end the perpetuation of the myth that teaching only occurs when the patient is in bed. Many good practicing physicians give more time to their outpatients than their inpatients, and they are no less sophisticated in their under-standing of disease because of their approach. The magnitude of the revolution of attitudes that is required in medical education to achieve these ends is hard to overestimate. When all patients receive a complete data base, when all records are problem-oriented, and when progress notes on each problem from its faintest beginning are available and audited, the folly of our present approaches will be even more apparent. The complete list of problems will be used as often to tell us when to stop futile activity in a ward as it will to tell us when to start profitable action in the clinic. As we now function with populations that are not defined and records that are kept at random, we stray further and further from good manage-ment principles as we frantically try to deal with health emergen-cies. Approaches that are truly humanitarian in the largest sense require that we be leaders who prevent problems, instead of follow-ers who take false pride in solving them.

LACK OF CONTINUITY OF CARE

Lack of continuity of care by the same physician is associated with doctors in training and specialists in medical centers and urban areas to a far greater degree than it is with the community physician with a relatively stable practice. In one urban clinic, more than two-thirds of the patients did not receive the continuity of care that comes from a single case being followed by a single physician.* The consequences in both patient and physician confusion and

* Marvin B. Sussman, *et. al., The Walking Patient: A Study in Outpatient Care,* Cleveland, The Press of Case Western Reserve University, 1967.

disorder are easy to conjecture. Tests may be repeated unnecessarily, results may not be followed up, and large amounts of time may be wasted by physician and patient, even when records are already adequate. A physician familiar with a complete, highly structured, problem-oriented medical record kept by himself can make sound judgments and decisions in a fraction of the time that a physician unfamiliar with the record requires.

BASIC SCIENCE TRAINING, THE PHYSICIAN, AND THE MEDICAL RECORD

If through the patient's record we can transmit some of the precepts of good scientific training in the clinical years, what should we expect in the preclinical years? Surely the basis of whatever we achieve during these years is absolute honesty. Students have a right to know that a great deal that they learn—Krebs' cycle, phage genetics, or membrane theory—cannot at the present time be applied by them (or often by anyone) directly to the complex biological problems that will confront them. It should also be admitted that simply the quantity of molecular biology and theoretical physiology that is now developing can frustrate and overwhelm anyone if it is not coordinated with his research or his continuing development, and that many basic scientists teaching in medical schools "find it more interesting to explore the fascinating interactions of genetics and chemistry in their uniquely favorable 'non-clinical' material than to bother about 'correlations with' medical and other practical matters."* Furthermore, the infinite elaboration of details in the laboratory of the basic scientist seems frequently to lead him away from the clinician instead of toward him.

The student correctly asks: "Can basic sciences be meaningfully related to my future?" It should be clearly pointed out to him that details oriented to specific problems and recorded in an organized manner in clinical records can do much to make correlations between basic science facts and clinical problems possible, but in addition each generation of physicians must learn basic science facts not

* F. M. Burnet, "Genetics of Microorganisms," *British Medical Bulletin,* 18:1, 1962.

yet applicable and carry them forward to the clinical years so that they themselves may discover the unexplored correlations that surely are there. Medical students are a crucial link between basic science and medical practice, since their clinical elders fall behind in basic science and technology, and their Ph. D. basic science elders do not know the clinical problems so that obvious correlations escape them. Until medical students visualize themselves as this fundamental link in a chain of progress instead of as passive receptacles of established wisdom, they will never assume the creative, constructive role that they alone can fill.

Basic science training must contribute to clinical performance through the teaching of systematic approaches. The physician as a preclinical student must be required by the basic scientist to formulate problems and write protocols as well as perform experiments. It is the capacity to formulate and pursue a problem that distinguishes a good clinician. A teacher of basic science has failed the physician if he does not impart this discipline but merely dispenses facts through lectures and standard experiments. Patients do not appear accompanied by a convenient syllabus and therapeutic plan.

There is one fundamental aspect in the preparation of the physician which the basic scientist is not prepared to teach. Basic scientists are themselves taught to choose and focus on a single problem or a limited number of problems, and they teach neither the philosophy nor the techniques for coping with the multiplicity of problems that patients inevitably present. The failure of clinical teachers to develop and articulate an approach to multiple problems has led to a serious discontinuity in the scientific training of the physician. The chaotic medical record is a symptom of this philosophical blind spot. The degree to which we organize the record and elevate it to the level of a scientific document will be a measure of our capacity to develop and teach a workable philosophy of multiple problems.

MEDICAL ROUNDS AND CONFERENCES

Years ago, when bedside and autopsy-table teaching predominated, most of the data used in medical discussions were acquired at the bedside. The bed was therefore a powerful mechanism to keep physicians and students anchored to the realities of their patient's problems. At present, even though some teaching at the bedside has continued, the collection of data is no longer done exclusively by the physician, and discussion has frequently become ritualistic, taking place from memory and at random rather than from highly organized, problem-oriented manuscripts. Ritual is a positive deterrent to rational progress in total patient care. No good scientist would make a judgment or even a recommendation on a single oral presentation of data; neither would he fail to follow up the result of his judgment. When they deal with serious problems, scientists study their data carefully before discussing them with anyone. No scientist would seriously consider medical rounds, as frequently conducted, good science, good care, or good education. Only through the availability for study by physicians and students of well-organized, problem-oriented records can recollected and refined medical judgments be developed.

The availability of such records could be the basis for a major change in teaching rounds. Rounds conducted on the basis of problem-oriented records do, of course, require that the attending physician study the data beforehand; time that is now spent presenting cases, establishing the basic sequence of care, and displaying random erudition would be spent instead analyzing and criticizing and redirecting the recorded efforts of the physician in solving the patient's problems. The young physician should be taught to anticipate and indeed enjoy such analyses for the rest of his life.

We should be allowed the luxury of conferences, grand rounds, or a clinical pathological conference only when the original data are in good order and completely and carefully presented. Ideally, copies of the complete, problem-oriented record should be delivered to every participant before the conference, but until computerization and easy facsimile reproduction make that possible, problem-oriented summaries at least should be prepared. An example of such a summary, prepared by Dr. D. Starbuck while he was an intern at the Cleveland Metropolitan General Hospital, is presented in Appendix C.

It should be noted, however, that certain educational goals cannot be met even by problem-oriented summaries and the well-ordered rounds and conferences for which they are prepared. Summaries, containing only selected data, are not sufficient for rigorous analysis and medical education. The goal in teaching is to guide the physician in the most effective development and application of his own resource of factual information through his own disciplined study of actual cases. The computer can make an enormous contribution in this area. Problem-oriented medical records can be made easily accessible to authorized individual physicians or participants in medical conferences who then can be expected to study patient data and analyze the list of problems, the plans, and the progress notes.*

MEANINGFUL AUDIT

The proper numbering and titling of progress notes makes it possible to appraise, through auditing, the quality of data, analysis, and medical performance in any one of the patient's problems, major or minor. The four premises of a problem-oriented audit of the physician can be stated as:

Premise 1. All the data in the medical record must be associated with a specific problem in order to determine whether the data are fundamental to solving the problem and whether factors such as redundancy, unnecessary delay, and lapse in judgment are present.

Premise 2. All the data on any given problem must be easily retrieved in sequence and with complete currency (i.e., X ray and laboratory data must be in the record as soon as they are available), so that the staff member responsible in a given specialty area for determining whether certain standards for quality are being met can make an accurate assessment. At the outset, the staff member will use the same criteria he has always used to assess the quality of

---

* At the Cleveland Metropolitan General Hospital, the computer aspects of such developments are being investigated under the direction of Mr. Jan Schultz.

management in his area. Eventually, as the data bank grows in both number of patients with a given problem and numbers of variables followed and recorded, new standards for reasonable numbers of tests and good care will emerge.

Premise 3. Standards for quality of patient care as outlined in premise 2 may evolve easily when a patient has a single problem or several unrelated problems. *Conclusions will be much more difficult when there are concomitant problems in the same patient* (cardiac failure, renal failure, malnutrition, etc.), the final solution of any one of which is intimately related to the progress on the others. *In these particular cases fixed standards of care do not apply, and quality must be determined individually,* within a framework of generally accepted principles. The doctor's role in cases of this type may well be likened to that of an analogue computer that plots specific points on a curve as a function of the time and type of input but does not establish the final shape of the curve until the input stops.

Premise 4. The dimensions of the quality control problem alluded to in Premises 2 and 3 can never be assessed until computerization of the data is accomplished. Manual approaches have not, after all these years, resulted in a widely applicable and practical approach. It is through their employment in rapid, effective audits and the corresponding demand for explicitness in the definition of problems and the orderly organization of the data that computers can make their main contribution to improving the performance and accelerating the professional development of physicians. Physicians will be able to govern their own professional advance to the degree that they are provided with comprehensive representations of what they have done to meet specific problems.

10

COMPUTERIZATION OF THE MEDICAL RECORD

Every phase of medical action will benefit from computerization. The "data base" phase can profit immediately. As stated earlier, the published work of Slack *et al.* and Mayne and Wedsel* has demonstrated the feasibility of employing the computer as a tool for obtaining a complete "systems review" of every patient by his direct interaction with a TV-type terminal that is the point of computer input. That input, structured by the computer, can be printed out in ordinary language and in narrative form for the physician's use.

Manual methods of recording medical history and performing systems review present many problems: owing to the time limitations faced by the physician, histories are often incomplete; the lengthy routine of history-taking utilizes physician skills that could

* W. B. Slack, G. P. Hicks, C. E. Reed, and L. J. Van Cura, "Computer-Based Medical-History System," *New England Journal of Medicine*, 274:194, 1966; J. G. Mayne and W. Wedsel, "Automating the Medical History," *Mayo Clinic Proceedings*, 43 (1):1, 1968.

more profitably be spent in performing other, more sophisticated functions; the historical portion of the patient's data base is the result of a single encounter by a single physician with a single individual, and the inevitable eccentricity of each encounter detracts from the accuracy and reproducibility of the information that it has provided; the absence of any formal standard for the minimum required data base allows many variations in the quality of the information elicited; the simple illegibility of many traditional histories makes the retrieval of information for patient care and research very difficult.

Recent experimentation with new techniques in the field of medical data acquisition has utilized digital computers to format and print-out patient responses to a set of medical-historical questions. Both self-administered and interviewer-administered questionnaires have been used, the latter feeding into the computer through an optical-scan reader. Medical histories produced by these methods (1) have a clearly defined content, independent of physician interest, time, and competence, because each patient is asked the same set of questions and can take as long as desired in answering; (2) do not require any expenditure of physician time; (3) give responses which can be checked by the physician to insure accuracy; (4) guarantee a minimum data base for the reasons given in (1); and (5) are legible owing to their reproduction as print-out rather than script.

Both self-administered and interviewer-administered questionnaires have significantly reinforced the quality of the data base. In our studies at the Cleveland Metropolitan General Hospital, a comparison of physician histories with those printed out by the computer revealed that significant information was being omitted by physicians in so-called complete work-ups. At the same time, an initial interviewer-computer approach in which the computer was used simply to register information failed to elicit the desired data base because, as positive findings arose, it proved extremely difficult to pursue them in sufficient depth through the employment of appropriate branching sub-questions, introduced into the individual protocol of questions in response to such positive findings. We concluded that this progressive refinement through successively more explicit sub-questions could not realistically be provided using "yes-no" sheets or IBM cards keyed by the interviewer and read by the computer.

It has proved possible, however, to provide appropriate branching questions through the use of a television screen (cathode-ray display console) and a computer program that does display sub-questions when they are triggered by a particular response to a more general question. The patient's response to the general question is analyzed by the computer, and additional questions programmed for that particular response are then shown. Slack and co-workers, in the article cited above, have demonstrated the feasibility of this method. No intermediary data exchange between the patient and the computer is required. The high-speed branching capabilities of the computer enable a dialogue to take place in which the questions asked become a continuing function of the patient's response to earlier questions.

In some similar systems the number of responses has been limited to four, each made by pushing a button. Present efforts at the Cleveland Metropolitan General Hospital employ a display console, developed by the Control Data Corporation, which allows ten choices by the patient in response to each question. The choice is made by the patient's physically touching the desired response displayed on the screen. When the patient interview has been completed, a print-out, by body system, of the patient's responses in ordinary language and in a narrative format is produced by the computer.

Each patient's responses are also retained in a "response file" in the computer memory. Interrogation of this file permits evaluation of the questions asked at a particular point in the history of the system, both in terms of desired medical knowledge and the factor of patient comprehension. Modifications in the individual history may be made as the result of this evaluation, and the content of the past medical history and systems review is therefore dynamic, the final goal being the formulation of a minimum data base for good comprehensive medical care.

Since these data on each patient are held by the computer, the potential exists for performing a much easier and more accurate health-hazard appraisal on each individual. It will be possible to inform him of actions he can take to reduce risk of disease. This possibility is contingent upon and related to epidemiological studies, which will themselves be greatly facilitated by the system, since the raw data will already be available in an easily manipulated form.

Every patient can thus be guaranteed a minimal recorded data base of historical information routinely acquired by his interaction with an organized, computer-administered series of branching questions. The doctor will always be expected to audit this information, enlarge upon it where indicated, and integrate it with information he himself has elicited. In this way recorded historical data will no longer narrowly be based on a single encounter, and busy physicians, representing a wide spectrum of abilities, habits of thoroughness, attitudes, and levels of efficiency, will not risk the omission of important problems.

Appendix A contains the initial set of questions developed for the purposes described above.* As experience grows and results are analyzed, new questions will be added and some old ones no doubt deleted. These questions are presented as a beginning point for students and other workers, and in no way are they to be construed as the best possible set for the establishment of a sound data base for the formulation of all of the patient's problems.

The statement of present illness and the progress notes, usually related in an unstructured manner, are the portions of the medical record that present the greatest difficulty in computerization. Although it has been awkward and too time-consuming to ask enough simple "yes-no" questions to obtain the desired record and then to print-out responses in narrative form, it has been possible to tie together logical choices from displays appearing in rapid succession on the TV-like screen. For example, the physician is first asked to identify the body system appropriate to the patient's present illness or identify the specific problem when writing a progress note. He is

---

* Stephen Cantrill of the Cleveland Metropolitan General Hospital, who prepared the material in the appendix, also prepared this discussion of it.

then confronted with a display containing the common symptoms presented in diseases of that particular system or displays containing the appropriate and up-to-date choices for the analysis and management of a specific problem. For example:

GASTROINTESTINAL

Jaundice	Dysphagia
Pain	Anorexia
Sore throat and/or mouth	Bleeding mouth or gums
Gassiness	Abnormal stools
Hiccuping	Vomiting

The physician indicates his choice of a symptom by touching it with his finger where it appears in the display on the screen. The next frame, which is displayed immediately and automatically on the screen, asks whether the symptom was gradual or sudden in onset. In like manner, a rapid succession of displays appears in which the following characteristics of the symptoms are presented:

Type of onset
When symptom commenced
Intensity
Quality
Severity
Location
Radiation
Number of episodes
Length of episodes
Time of episodes
Relieved by
Made worse by
Associated with
Course—getting better, getting worse, staying the same

The frame displayed for each characteristic contains from two to ten choices, and if the number of descriptive choices makes it necessary, two frames are used in rapid succession for a given characteristic. The "type of onset" frame contains two choices, for example, whereas the "associated with" frame may contain ten or more, depending upon the symptom.

These frames not only provide a consistent, logical means for entering the present illness and progress notes but also are effective teachers of the physician. They continually call to mind a range of symptomatic characteristics, with regard, for instance, to abdominal pain, that will be the foundation of a sound diagnosis. These frames should be developed and approved by experts in each field, so that every patient gets the benefit of a high sophistication in the formulation of the branching series of questions employed in exploring his particular complaint, regardless of his particular physician's experience, specialty, and capacity for analysis. This approach, it will be observed, is based on recognition, as opposed to recall, and thereby introduces consistency and thoroughness into every performance. Similar displays have been developed for objective data (Fig. 8).

Below is an example of a statement of present illness written in the conventional manner and a statement of the same present illness prepared using the TV-like terminal with sequential displays developed, in this case, by Dr. Philip Guzelian in association with staff members of the Cleveland Metropolitan General Hospital.

Statement of Present Illness, Prepared in a Conventional Manner

The patient was in his usual state of fair health until four months prior to admission when he noticed the onset of periodic vomiting and hiccuping. Initially both problems were not associated with or precipitated by any specific activity. The patient did, however, note the presence of diffuse abdominal pain which was most intense in the epigastric region, which radiated into the flank regions and which he described as a deep, hard pain. When present the pain was constant without variation in intensity and was noted to last for variable periods of time, occasionally as long as all day or all night. The patient states that the pain was ameliorated somewhat by taking Dristan and initially by the ingestion of food. Three weeks prior to admission, however, the patient states that he caught the flu, manifested by the sudden onset of shaking chills followed by a fever which remained up until the time of admission. Associated with the onset of flu his vomiting increased in frequency and was apparently related to the ingestion of food or fluid. The patient states that he was unable to keep anything down. Abdominal pain was aggravated by vomiting which the patient describes as projective (a distance of three feet?). The patient notes 50 lb. (210 to 154) weight loss three months prior to admission.

Statement of Present Illness, Prepared by use of a TV-Like Terminal

VOMITING commencing 4 months ago. Repeated episodes. Times of episodes, immediately P.C. [after meals] but any time day or night. Severity, moderate amount. Quality, whitish, projectile, non-projectile. Associated with weight loss, abdominal pain, drinking alcoholic beverages, flu or infection, fever and regurgitation. Getting worse.

HICCUPING commencing 4 months ago. Did not determine intensity. Repeated episodes. Lasting variable periods. Did not determine episode time. Made worse by nothing. Associated with weight loss, regurgitation. Getting worse.

PAIN commencing 4 months ago. Did not determine type of onset. Moderate intensity. Repeated episodes lasting hours. Quality, deep. Location, epigastric. Radiating to flank region. Associated with weight loss, regurgitation. Relieved by food. Made worse by food.

Some information in the first version is not represented in the second, for example, the patient's use of Dristan. Peculiar detail of this kind may, by use of the typewriter keyboard that is part of the TV-like terminal, be specially entered by the physician into the patient's record. Or, if the information omitted is more general in nature and may be expected to be of value to the physician either currently or for prospective studies, the standard displays may be altered so as to include it. In the illustration above, for example, the original display should have asked for exact increment or decrement of weight. A corresponding alteration in the displays was promptly made. Conversely, when displays prove in time to be defective, they may be removed.

It will be noted in the example above that the phrase "did not determine" appears. On all displays the physician must either choose descriptors or enter his failure to make such a determination. This method assures that the data will be reliable for clinical investigative studies as well as for current care, since failure to enter is always recorded as a positive act. It will also be noted that phrases appear which seem contradictory, e.g., "relieved by food" and "made worse by food." By such apparent contradictions the computer indicates that over time both characteristics are true, that is, that at times food relieved the symptom and at times seemed to make it worse.

Displays are easily modified in terms of sequence of content. For example, some clinicians prefer to isolate general symptoms, such

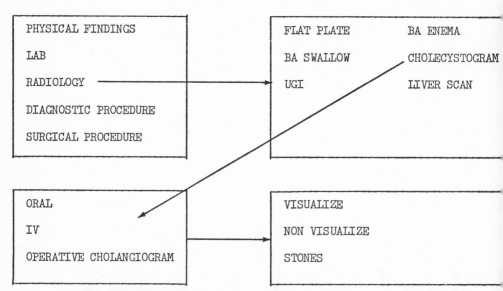

FIGURE 8. Computer displays developed for objective data. (IV = intravenous; UGI = upper gastrointestinal series.)

as weight loss, fatigability, fever, and malaise, and to locate them in advance of the detailed analysis of any one symptom. This sequence avoids redundancy and also reveals in one short paragraph the over-all constitutional effects of an illness. There is evidence that such a method is useful in prognosis, particularly with certain types of malignancy.

The initial response of many physicians to highly structured standards for the description of symptoms is a degree of doubt and concern. They suspect that delicacy of description is absent from such standards, and indeed the accounts prepared in accordance with the standards do seem to show a certain sameness of expression. In reality, however, the possible combinations of symptoms, descriptions, and times are practically limitless. Each account is unique, though phases within accounts do recur—much as each chess game is different though a limited "vocabulary" of spaces and chessmen is used. This rich variety of possible combinations of identical phrases is the very characteristic that makes objective data so attractive and useful to the physician. Rarely does the physician discard his objective data in favor of random, expressionistic descriptions of the same phenomena. The rejection of standardization of "language" on the one hand in the name of art, and the acceptance of order on the other in the name of science have led to a failure in our profession to exploit rigorously much valuable symptomatic information. Physicians' attitudes toward standard descriptors can be altered if computerized approaches to symptomatic data continue to show practical benefits and if the profession comes to realize that the word "art" was never meant to be applied to undisciplined, casual accounts that omit crucial descriptors and add others that are reported in such personal terms that they have a different meaning for every reader. The true "art" lies in the imaginative interpretation of and action upon multiple variables that are consistently defined and accurately analyzed and transmitted.

This approach is being facilitated by the work of Dr. Burgess Gordon, of the American Medical Association, who is revising current medical terminology to reduce the number of terms for a single disease and the multiplicity of descriptors and qualifiers. The pioneering work of Dr. Morris Collen,* as well, in studying many variables in hundreds of thousands of patients will help the physician to choose those that are most pertinent to the identification and management of the largest number of important medical problems.

In addition to the narrative information constituting the data base, logic would seem to indicate that statements of problems should be entered into the computer. Study at Cleveland Metropolitan General Hospital, after analysis of large numbers of manually recorded problems, has demonstrated the feasibility of using logically grouped displays of problems and the general system described above. That is, the physician makes a choice on the TV-like terminal and, in some situations, is led through further displays requiring more careful delineation of the problem. For example, he is first required to state whether the problem in a given organ system is a "diagnosis," a physiological finding (such as heart failure), or a symptom or a laboratory finding (such as abnormal electrocardiogram). If he chooses heart failure he will be required in the next display, which appears automatically, to say whether compensated or decompensated, biventricular, right side or left. These previously prepared displays enable easy encoding and yet give freedom of expression to the physician. This method is a tacit teacher because it requires the physician to formulate his problems consistently, completely, and accurately.

The role of the computer in a diagnosis or, what is more appropriate to our discussion, formulation of the problems has been the subject of study by many investigators.** Easy success in applying

* M. F. Collen, L. Rubin, and L. Davis, "Computers in Multiphasic Screening," in *Computers in Biomedical Research*, New York, Academic Press, 1965, Chapter 14.
** R. Ledley and L. Lusted, "Reasoning Foundations of Medical Diagnosis," *Science*, 130.9, 1959; K. Brodman, "Diagnostic Decisions by Machine," *IRE Transactions on Medical Electronics*, ME-7:216, 1960; H. R. Warner, A. F. Toronto, and L. G. Veasy, "Experience with Bayes' Theorem for Computer Diagnosis of Congenital Heart Disease," *Annals of the New York Academy of Sciences*, 115:558, 1964; B. Kleinmuntz, "Clinical Information Processing," *Datamation*, 11:41, 1965; F. J. Moore, "Concept of a Clinical Decision Support System," IBM Advanced Systems Development Division Technical Report, 1966.

the computer to diagnostic problems was not to be expected and has not been achieved for several reasons. The word "diagnosis" is in itself ambiguous. We call an ulcer a diagnosis and a fever a symptom when neither term is clearly understood. Mathematics, and particularly Bayesian theory, has not been as helpful as one might have hoped because patients inconveniently do not provide either single or mutually exclusive problems, nor do physicians show consistency either in behavior or in the quality of the data they employ. Furthermore, physicians randomly mix data collection and therapeutic action and thereby create new problems that defy traditional methods of analysis. The need for and value of help at the strictly diagnostic level has also been to some degree overrated. Rational management is often based on the physiological state of the patient, as measured by standard parameters, and not on any categorical etiological diagnosis. The quantitative aspects of disease in terms of criticality and severity frequently determine therapy, and they are not always implicit in the simple statement of the diagnosis.

What course of action should be followed in the face of the above difficulties? We should use modern computer techniques as described here and by others as well as all available resources of modern technology to make the initial data base as large as possible. "Diagnosis" is frequently obvious if all the data are available initially. A consultant's expertise consists often of little more than organizing a crucial element of the information already available, so that the true nature of the problem becomes obvious. Modern techniques can provide a "synthetic" expertise of this type as they record and present massive amounts of data in closely logical form. Gradually the computer will help the physician to become an intelligent "guidance system" by grouping certain abnormal findings and by directing the physician to obtain specific additional data as abnormalities appear. Understanding therefore will come securely in small steps. The recorded data in medicine and the relevant mathematical techniques are simply not available at this time to permit the massive quantum leap from a few symptoms to the hypothetical world of diagnosis—nor need they be for the intelligent, effective management of patients.

All laboratory, X ray, and pharmacologic data will be ordered under a particular problem number and not merely under the patient's name and unit number. All results, as soon as they are available, will be printed in the records under the appropriate problem heading. Moreover, the entry of medication orders through a TV-type terminal affords an excellent opportunity to educate the physician. For example, in the future when a physician in the experimental system at the Cleveland Metropolitan General Hospital uses the terminal to order treatment for a problem, say hypertension, he will immediately be confronted with a display of the four or five antihypertensive agents in use in his institution. After choosing one of the drugs, reserpine for example, the physician will immediately see a series of displays related to reserpine (see Fig. 9). The first frame emphasizes cautions or even contra-indications to the drug's use, while the subsequent frames outline common side effects, specify usual dosages, and present relevant information regarding mechanism of action, metabolism, and excretion—if these are known. Finally a frame will appear by means of which the physician can actually order the drug. In this way pharmacologic information, both observed and theoretical, is linked directly to patient care. This factor of relevance is fundamental to efficient education. By presenting both factual and theoretical information, the physician's basic knowledge is enhanced and he is made aware of new developments in clinical pharmacology. As the physician's knowledge of drugs is enlarged he should be better able to deliver appropriate, and safe, therapy to the patient.*

There is considerable urgency in this matter of the computerization of medical records. Already large amounts of money have been allocated to the computerization of single components in the hospital complex—laboratories, pharmacies, etc.—with little regard to the

---

* The procedure described above was developed through the efforts of Dr. George Nelson, Cleveland Metropolitan General Hospital. Of course such a format requires frequent review so that the data presented are current and accurate. A procedure whereby the various subspecialties periodically review the literature and update related drug information would be a logical means of acquiring this currency.

orientation of data to patient problems. This proliferation of auto-mated systems within parts of a hospital complex without provision for a central focus on patient problems makes evaluation of all these expensive efforts difficult. Such automation may result in highly efficient and accurate specific tests and maneuvers, but in many instances it may also merely be facilitating rapid action in those special areas without affecting the solution of the patient's problems. Daily reporting of an accurate chemistry value, for example, has no particular virtue if the problem at hand requires only a weekly determination or no such determination at all. Laboratories have proceeded on the assumption that all determi-nations that are ordered are indicated and that the frequency of given determinations is never excessive. Major investments have been made in systems that were never designed to test this crucial and questionable assumption.

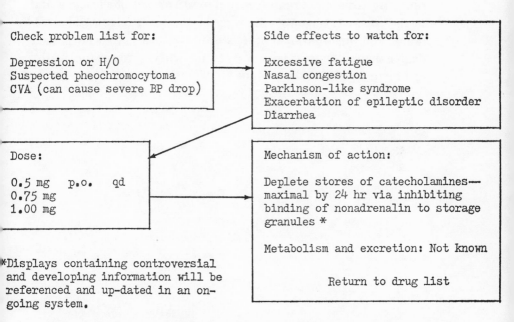

FIGURE 9. Displays following the choice of the drug reserpine. (H/O = history of; CVA = cerebrovascular accident; BP = blood pressure; p.o. = by mouth; qd = daily.)

At the present time no operational system exists that permits a medical teacher or member of an accrediting agency to take a patient's record at random, select one of the patient's problems, review all the data pertinent to that problem in sequence, and so assess whether current medical standards are being properly applied. Also at the present time the details of the relationship between patient's problems and hospital resources and costs are very obscure. A medical record maintained by the technique described will make possible a fiscal management in which specific utilization of medical resources and services for the care of the patient, problem by problem, is a matter of the medical record. It will enable the hospital to establish a dynamic unit-cost-accounting system similar to that employed by more sophisticated industries. The advantages of such a system have broad and favorable implications for the general management of health-care systems in the areas of fiscal planning, organization of resources, and measurement of efficiency, and in the effective, ongoing education of medical students. The economic and organizational aspects of medical care, to a far greater degree than students are presently aware, will determine the quality and quantity of care they will be able to deliver.

11

MEDICAL
RESPONSIBILITY

The justification for a reorganization of the medical record by identifying all data with a specific problem is not based, and cannot by the nature of the case be based, on any proof that the reorganization will in itself guarantee improved quality of care and education. Bibliographies of literatures, complex classification systems in organic chemistry, and well-established rules for presenting data in scientific manuscripts do not guarantee the quality of the data that are being regulated, and no one expects them to, in and of themselves. But order is certainly conducive to quality, and it would be unthinkable for a serious scholar to study a literature, take up a problem in organic chemistry or referee technical manuscripts if he first were required to accept a mass of incomplete and randomly presented basic data and organize it, before even approaching the matter of quality in a particular case. It is hard for nonmedical scientists to believe that we physicians have for so long allowed chaos to exist in everyday medical data; since scientists are not usually engaged in the study of several problems simultaneously as doctors are, scientists are more easily able to proceed to the qualitative evaluation of their discrete areas of interest. Physicians thus far have not developed a system for maintaining progress notes on several problems simultaneously. However difficult the problem of order is to them, they must nevertheless come to regard the creation of methods for organizing the record as the basis for any program of quality control in medicine.

If there is no adequate record of what a doctor does and what he fails to do, how can the quality of the care he provides be assessed? There are residents and staff physicians who maintain that the content of their records ought properly to be their concern alone. In reality, however, it is the patient's concern and the concern of those who in the future will have to depend on those records for the continuing care of the patient or for medical research. There are physicians who say they do not have the time to maintain complete, problem-oriented records. They should be reminded that the prompt, orderly registration of data is the only basis for an ultimate efficiency in the application of their professional resources that is going to save time and lives.

Failure to keep accurate and up-to-date records may be regarded as a form of secrecy. When a physician restricts the knowledge of his art to himself by keeping unintelligible records, he may be denying his patient the illumination that is his right. Indian medicine men and ancient Egyptian priests guarded their secrets to keep uninformed and fearful patients in their grip. The failure to create the kind of medical record that will tell everyone authorized to know exactly what a physician has done is an analogous form of secrecy— and secrecy has no place in the science of medical practice.

THE RESPONSIBILITY FOR TOTAL CARE

Implicit in much of what has been said here about care of the patient, education of the physician, and preparation of proper medical records is the assumption that total care should be provided to all individuals and that resources are sufficient to cover the whole population in such a manner. It is not known whether this assumption is correct. We could proceed as if it were, work conscientiously on an ideal model of total care, and attempt to extend it rapidly to all. We could, on the other hand, proceed as if resources are inadequate to provide total medical care for all and therefore make it a matter of priority to collect a minimum, but nevertheless defined, data base on the whole population, screening rapidly for gross and principal medical/surgical problems such as hypertension, diabetes, obvious cancer, heart disease, severe psychiatric disease, and common, correctible surgical disorders. We could, equipped with this data base, set up facilities to provide for all the simplest forms of effective treatment of such gross problems. Such an approach has been applied to tuberculosis, for example. Having secured this much care for the total population, we could then do as academic medicine has traditionally done and concern ourselves intensively with uncommon disorders, such as rare metabolic diseases or unusual surgical transplant procedures.

We should not preach total care and then fail to practice it. To do so is unworthy of our science. It is easy to talk in fashionable terms about comprehensive care, family care, and neighborhood health centers and then in practice to ignore broad social and medical obstacles, to neglect most of the data base necessary to apply such concepts, to treat chief complaints only, and to plan for continuing care and follow up patients carelessly if at all.

There need be no compromise on the first phase of medical action—obtaining a data base on everyone. Modern technology has made this phase completely feasible, whether judged on the basis of the economic or the personnel demands it would be likely to make, and the physician shortage cannot be used as an argument against it. There are good reasons to separate this initial phase from the others, at least as the universal data base is being built, so that those obtaining the base are not expected to (and need not ever be able to) formulate or treat problems. There is no reason to doubt, in other words, that paramedical personnel could be the chief human instruments in the creation of the universal base.

Once such a base had been created, its effects upon the organization and application of medical resources, though conjectural, would be likely to be profound, and profoundly promising. Levels of patient problems could be selected for solution. Priorities could be established, so that certain problems were treated only if resources allowed. Also, a complete data base removes the risk of treating problems out of context. For example, it is possible that awareness of one problem (severe renal disease) would contraindicate action on another one (valvular lesion), even though data on the former were not obtained with the idea that available resources would be likely to permit its treatment. Given the universal data base, the computer would be of great assistance in designating patients for specialists on the basis of specific findings without permitting patient problems to become enmeshed in subtleties of diagnosis. Such designation, I suspect, would identify and mobilize the interests of the specialist and the profession as a whole to a surprising degree. Rational, humane medical care is after all what we all seek. It is true that many problems outside of the specialist's area of interest are always present in a given patient, but if the specialist's competence were shown to be immediately relevant to the principal problem of the patient I do not doubt that the specialist would respond. It may well be that with proper organization of the record and with the help of well-conceived problem-oriented computer displays he would find it possible to give reasonable attention to other problems as well. All physicians want to see patients in whom they have taken a special interest receive complete care, but many specialists quite understandably prefer not to undertake the responsibility for total care in patients who offer no opportunity for the practice of a hard-won expertise.

Further to project, a scheme of data collection sites and neighborhood and specialized health centers could be developed to administer and apply the resource of the universal data base. Data collection sites would, of course, gather the data base. Patients with minor or easily managed problems could be directed to neighborhood health centers; unusual and complex problems requiring specialized talent and equipment could be treated in a few specialized centers. All three segments in this health scheme—data collection sites, neighborhood health centers, and specialized health centers—would be united by a computerized record system, so that in no area would a problem be dealt with in ignorance or out of context.

I may be charged with romanticism or utopianism in suggesting, even so briefly, that the universal data base holds such implications. The projections I make are indeed far from the present *reality*, but they are not so far from the present *possibility*, and in this difference between reality and possibility there lies, I believe, a lesson for responsible physicians. Some may point to the obstacles that are created by the expectations of the patient himself: immediate physician contact with attention directed to symptoms and current conventional therapy (the "shot of penicillin"). But patients want what we have taught them to want through careless medical practices. If they want only hasty, symptomatic relief, then the answer is not to accede to that demand but patiently to educate the patient to the necessity of something better. It has been my experience that with little effort patients do come to understand the concepts of "the physician as a guidance system dependent on follow-up," a "complete data base," and "problems out of context" as well as physicians do—better, perhaps, than physicians who use "unreasonable" patient demands to justify their own lack of system and failure to educate the public.

IN CONCLUSION

One cannot survey the details of what physicians have done in the past and what they are doing now without wondering what the future holds for the art and science of medical practice and scholarly biological research. To the extent that art is discipline and form—as can be seen in the meter and rhyme of the poet's line or in the meticulously chosen dynamics of the musician's composition—to this extent medicine has never been an art in the hands of most of us, and we debase the word itself when we apply it to the undisciplined and disorganized encounters that characterize many doctor-patient relationships. To the extent that scholarship and the foundation of our profession in research should provide us with an Olympian view of the significance and interrelationships of the medical problems we are trying to solve—to this extent the fields of biology and medicine can be said to have produced more brilliant technicians than thoughtful and creative scholars.

Patient interviews as we have conducted them, patient records as we have known them, conferences as we have stumbled through them—all must be given a better framework of discipline and form. This can be done through the creative use of modern means of precise and immediate communication. Until we accept the principle that great art does not exist in opposition to structuring and form but requires them, we will never be able to reap the great benefits that the electronic and computer age holds in store. What was precisely communicated on paper by Bach, faithfully performed by Casals, and captured in recordings by modern technology is now available to countless thousands. In the same way, medicine at its best can also be generalized and made available to all if, for each problem, the best current medical standards for defining and treating that problem are available by modern electronic means to each physician. And this aim can and should be achieved in such a way that, as the physician actually records his data and plans the treatments, the very communication tools he uses will have built into them the parameters of guidance and the currency of information he needs to define and solve problems. The best talent medicine has must be available to him through computer displays at the time he performs, because it is at the point of integrating knowledge and action that he needs help, not in learning the facts themselves.

I recognize that up-to-date and precise communication will not alone lead to the best in medical practice, any more than precisely transcribed music makes a great performer, but it is equally true that without precision and form much art can never be transmitted. There will always be individuals whose performance is superior in a total sense because of subtleties yet to be defined in medical practice, but for most patients the physician's "art" will be sufficient if they can be assured that their doctor is aware of the highest standards of medical practice and if he handles the data on their problems in a disciplined and orderly way.

There are a few who fear that rigid concentration on the patient's problems will emphasize only the physician's practical knowledge and development, creating a species of tradesman who, enslaved by the technical expertise of an era, will be unable to meet new situations in a changing world. But the approaches described in this book will demand of the practitioner, the faculty, and the student clarity of thought, a research-oriented attitude, and a willingness to apply first principles to the changing situations inherent in the infinite variety of combinations of interacting medical problems. Biological realities, honestly confronted, facilitate rather than hinder scientific advance. That confrontation *is* the art of medicine.

APPENDICES

APPENDICES

APPENDIX A

Questionnaire Used for
Obtaining Patient's
Medical History by Computer

The questionnaire that follows was developed by Stephen Cantrill at the Cleveland Metropolitan General Hospital (CMGH), in consultation with various subspecialists at CMGH and other hospitals and after careful review of the Kaiser Permanente questionnaire, the earlier versions of the CMGH questionnaire, and the questionnaire developed by J. F. Kanner and associates, Lexington, Kentucky. Intended for use by patients in self-administered computerized interviews, as described in Chapter 10, this questionnaire represents an initial attempt in the construction of a cathode-ray-tube-based, patient-administered past medical history and systems review. The questions in several sections of the questionnaire have been annotated to show the significance of a positive response. This annotation will enable the student to understand the value of the information elicited by each question. It is expected that the content of this questionnaire will undergo further refinement. The questionnaire has been included here so that it can serve as a focus for further work by others as well as ourselves on this aspect of data gathering, and to this end suggested modifications, additions, or excisions should be addressed to:

> Lawrence L. Weed, M.D.
> PROMIS Laboratories
> College of Medicine
> University of Vermont
> Burlington, Vermont 05401

The sections of the past medical history and systems review are presented in the following order:

Social Profile	Cardiovascular
Family History	Musculoskeletal
Infectious Diseases	Endocrine
Immunizations	Breast
Eye, Ear, Nose, and Throat	Gynecology (females only)
Dermatology-Allergy	Obstetrical (females only)
Dental	Genitourinary
Gastrointestinal	Neurology
Hematopoietic	Psychiatry
Respiratory	

For ease in presentation and understanding, only a simplified skeleton of the questionnaire is presented here. There is no difference in gross content between the simplified and complete questionnaires, but in actual practice more use is made of past responses in determining branching, in order to "personalize" the questionnaire to the individual patient.

The questions have been set up on a series of levels, each indentation to the right indicating the next greater level. The basic rule for the questions having a yes-or-no response is: If the question is answered yes, the patient continues on to the next question; if answered no, he continues on to the next question that appears on the same or lesser indentation level. For example, in the social profile if the patient answers yes to question 16, he is then asked question 17; if his answer is no, he is asked question 19. With regard to single-choice questions, making one choice will automatically take the patient to the next question. For example, in question 32 of the profile, any question will lead the patient immediately to question 33. With multiple-choice questions, several choices can be specified as the response to a single question. Question 33 is an example of this type: The patient can make as many choices from this list as he deems necessary. He is only referred to the next question if he chooses "done" or "none of these." This type of question is used when a response is desired to a long series of similar questions, none of which is likely to yield a frequent positive response. Combination shortens the time necessary to administer the questionnaire and avoids a point of possible patient frustration. For example, the first five questions of the family history are equivalent to 35 questions with a "yes-no" response.

Some items, such as rheumatic fever, have not been grouped with other similar choices, because of the position of particular importance they have assumed in the traditional practice of medicine.

Some questions are exceptions to the above general rules and have their own branching patterns. In such cases, each response is accompanied by the number of the question, in brackets, that will follow if that response is made. For example, if the question is followed by "Yes [Go to 27] No [Go to 24]," question 27 or 24 will next be asked, depending upon the patient's response.

Several questions appear more than once in the questionnaire. This duplication provides a validity check in general on the whole questionnaire as well as a check on several very important areas of inquiry.

After the questionnaire has been completed by the patient, the computer generates and prints-out the past medical history and the systems review by reporting only desired factual data (e.g., that the patient is a male) and "abnormal" responses (e.g., that the patient had syphilis is of interest and would be included; however, that he did *not* have syphilis would not be included). This "print-out by exception" (printing abnormal responses) requires that the physician have a working knowledge of the questionnaire if he is to take best advantage of the information presented in the print-out.

Although not included in the following list, each question has a "don't know" and "don't understand" response. If the patient should indicate the "don't understand" response he will receive assistance from an attendant. A "don't know" response will be noted as such and for purposes of branching will be considered a negative response.

The following is a brief example of the type of print-out produced by such a system.

MUSCULO-SKELETAL:

HAD DIFFICULTY PARTICIPATING IN SPORTS WHEN YOUNG. PROBLEMS WERE WITH COORDINATION. HAS HAD BROKEN ANKLE.
PAINFUL JOINTS ARE PRESENT AND PAST PROBLEM. JOINTS INVOLVED ARE KNEES. THERE HAS BEEN SWELLING AND HEAT IN THESE JOINTS.
HAS PAIN IN LOWER BACK. HAS HAD THIS FOR MORE THAN 6 MONTHS. PAIN IS GETTING WORSE.

The physician will then pursue these points in greater depth where necessary, the questionnaire having prevented significant omissions, thereby fulfilling the requirement of a minimum standardized data base.

The categorizations, as well as the content of the entire questionnaire, are subject to change as data derived from computerization provide the necessary insight and should be studied with this possibility of alteration in mind.

SOCIAL PROFILE

1. You will now be asked a series of questions about your past medical history. To answer each question, touch the box next to your answer on the TV screen.

   Do you have any questions?

   No [Go to 3]   Yes [Go to 2]

2. Please ask the interviewer for help. She will help you to understand.

3. I am a

   Male   Female

4. My age is about

   10 years to 19 years [Go to 5]   60 to 69 years
   20 to 29 years   70 to 79 years
   30 to 39 years   80 to 89 years
   40 to 49 years   90 to 99 years
   50 to 59 years

5. My age is exactly

   10 years ⎫   15 years ⎫
   11 years ⎪   16 years ⎪
   12 years ⎬ [Go to 6]   17 years ⎬ [Go to 6]
   13 years ⎪   18 years ⎪
   14 years ⎭   19 years ⎭

   [Similar frames for other age ranges]

6. I was born in

Northeastern U.S.	Western U.S.
Eastern U.S.	Southwestern U.S.
Southern U.S.	Other than U.S.

7. The town I was born in was

Large (more than 50,000)
Medium (more than 5,000 but less than 50,000)
Small (less than 5,000 but more than 100)
Rural (out in the country)

8. I have lived in the area where I now live for

all my life	6 to 9 years
40 years or more	3 to 5 years
30 to 39 years	1 to 2 years
20 to 29 years	less than one year
10 to 19 years	

9. In school I have graduated from the 8th grade.

Yes [Go to 11]   No [Go to 10]

10. The highest grade that I finished in school was

didn't go to ⎫	4th grade ⎫
school ⎪	5th grade ⎪
1st grade ⎬ [Go to 12]	6th grade ⎬ [Go to 12]
2nd grade ⎪	7th grade ⎪
3rd grade ⎭	8th grade ⎭

11. The highest grade that I finished in school was

8th grade ⎫	Technical School ⎫
9th grade ⎪	Junior College ⎪
10th grade ⎬ [Go to 12]	College ⎬ [Go to 13]
11th grade ⎭	Post Graduate ⎭
12th grade [Go to 13]	

12. I didn't continue in school because

school work was too difficult	of pregnancy
I didn't like school	of illness
I wanted to earn money	I had to help at home
	Some other reason

13. I would like to get further education.

14. I have been discouraged about trying to get more education.

15. I would like to talk to someone about this.

16. I would like to get on-the-job training.

17. I have been discouraged about trying to get training.

18. I would like to talk to someone about this.

19. I am married or have been married.

[If yes, skip to 22]

20. I live

alone
with my parents
with friends

with brothers or sisters
with other relatives

21. I have to cook my own meals.

[Skip to 31]

22. I am living with my spouse (with my husband or wife).

No [Go to 23]   Yes [Go to 24]

23. I live

alone
with my parents
with my brother or sister
with my children

with my grandchildren
with other relatives
with friends

[Go to 25]

24. I have been married more than once.

25. I am divorced.

26. It has happened within the past year.

[Skip to 31]

27. I am separated.

28. It has happened within the past year.

[Skip to 31]

29. I am widowed.

30. It has happened within the past year.

31. I have children who live with me and depend on me for support.

32. The number of these dependent children is

1 child	6 children
2 children	7 children
3 children	8 children
4 children	9 children
5 children	10 or more children

33. These are

my own children	adopted children
grandchildren	foster children
great grandchildren	none of these
done	

34. I have family or home problems with

my spouse (my husband or wife)	my children
	other relatives
my parents	neighbors
done	none of these

35. I would like to talk to someone about these problems.

36. I can depend on some of my friends or relatives to help me if I need it.

37. I have the responsibility for a relative or relatives.

38. I receive help or a member of my family receives help from the following social agencies:

Catholic Family and Children's Services	Jewish Family Service Association
	Juvenile Court
Child Guidance	Youth Services
Crippled Children's Services	other agency
	done or none of these
Family Service Association	

39. I am currently employed (I have a job).

    [If No, skip to 49]

40. I am employed

    full-time   part-time

41. I have

    1 job   2 jobs

42. I have had this present job for

    less than 1 year   4 years
    1 to 2 years   5 or more years
    3 years

43. I am satisfied with my present job.

44. I have difficulty holding my present job.

45. The main problem in holding my job is

    the other employees   my health
    my boss   other reasons

46. I would like to talk to someone about my present job or about getting a new job.

47. The physical activity I have on my job is best described as

    very active
    limited activity
    no physical activity (I sit at my job)

48. My job is best described as

    heavy labor   technical work
    a trade   food handling
    construction work   spot labor
    domestic work   professional
    sales or clerical work   other

                         [Skip to 51]

49. I have been unemployed

    a few days   one year
    a few weeks   2 years
    a few months   more than 2 years

50. The main reason that I am unemployed is
    my health   I can't find a job
    I don't want to work

51. I have financial problems that I would like to discuss with someone.

52. [Men] I have served in the armed forces.
                    [If yes or if woman, skip to 55]

53. I was rejected or deferred by the draft.

54. I was rejected or deferred
    for physical reasons
    for mental reasons
    because of my job or family

55. I have a home to go to today.

56. I have lived in my present home for
    less than 1 year   5 to 10 years
    1 to 2 years   more than 10 years
    3 to 5 years

57. The number of rooms I have in my house is
    1 room   4 rooms
    2 rooms   5 rooms
    3 rooms   more than 5 rooms

58. The number of bedrooms I have in my house is
    1 bedroom   3 bedrooms
    2 bedrooms   more than 3 bedrooms

59. The number of people who live in my house is
    1 person   7 people
    2 people   8 people
    3 people   9 people
    4 people   10 people
    5 people   more than 10 people
    6 people

60. In my home there is a place to take a bath.

61. In my home there is a place to take a shower.

62. In my home there is a place to wash myself.

63. I have to climb stairs in my home to get to the bathroom.

64. I have electric light in my home.

65. I have cooking facilities in my home.

66. I have enough heat in my home.

67. I am satisfied with my present housing.

68. I am planning to move this month or next.

69.   The reason I am moving is

    poor housing conditions . forced out by urban renewal
    eviction notice   other
    health

70. The amount of alcohol I drink is

    none [Go to 80]   a moderate amount
    a small amount   a large amount

71. I sometimes drink by myself.

72. I drink more now than I did last year.

73. I sometimes go on drinking sprees.

74. I sometimes cannot remember what I did while I was drinking.

75. I sometimes miss work on Monday morning.

76. I sometimes take a drink in the morning.

77. I need a drink before I can face certain situations.

78. I have been in the hospital because of drinking.

79. I have lost a job because of my drinking.

80. There has recently been a big change in my way of life.

81.   This change is related to

    my family
    my job
    my health

82. This change is for the better.

83. I eat 2 or more meals a day.

84. I have meat or eggs with one or more meals a day.

85. I often skip breakfast.

86. I often skip a noon meal.

87. I snack more than 3 times a day.

88. I have special food customs or beliefs.

89. I visit with friends or relatives frequently.

90. I sometimes attend
    church | community group meetings
    PTA meetings | meetings of other clubs or organi-
    done | zations
    | none of these

91. I have some legal problems that I would like to talk about.

92. I am currently engaged in a lawsuit.

93. I am currently getting medical or psychiatric care someplace else.

94. I see a doctor regularly for health checkups.

95. The last physical exam I had done by a doctor was
    within past 6 months | 2 to 5 years ago
    6 months to 1 year ago | greater than 5 years ago
    1 to 2 years ago

96. For medical care or advice, I normally go to
    no place | special health services in the com-
    private doctor | munity
    hospital clinic | minister
    emergency room | pharmacist
    city health center | neighbor or friend

97. I generally feel tired and have physical pain.

98. I take things other than medicine prescribed by a doctor to make me feel better.

99. Costs have kept me from getting care when I thought I needed it.

100. Transportation problems and distance have kept me from getting care when I thought I needed it.

101. I need a person to stay at my home to take care of someone when I go to get medical care.

102. I have been discouraged, fearful, or confused about medical care that I have had in the past.

103. I was afraid of what might be found by the doctor.

104. I was confused because nobody explained anything to me.

105. I dislike the discourtesy I experienced.

106. The people where I was treated were not kind.

107. I drive a car.

108. I wear a seatbelt when I drive or ride in a car.

109. I sometimes take unnecessary risks as a pedestrian.

110. I own or often shoot a gun (includes rifles).

111. I know how to swim.

112. I am exposed to dangerous sources of fire or explosion.

113. I always take the proper precautions when exposed to these dangers.

114. I am currently taking or should be taking medicine.

FAMILY HISTORY

1. I have blood relatives who have had

anemia	arthritis
apoplexy or stroke	none of these
done	

2. I have blood relatives who have had

asthma or hay fever	alcoholism
bleeding tendency	cancer
cataracts	cirrhosis
color blindness	congenital heart disease
done	none of these

3. I have blood relatives who have had

diabetes	deafness before they were 50
eczema	epilepsy
emphysema	glaucoma
gout	heart disease
high blood pressure	high cholesterol
done	none of these

4. I have blood relatives who have had

insanity	kidney disease
kidney stones	leukemia
lung trouble	mental retardation
migraine headaches	nervous breakdown
done	none of these

5. I have blood relatives who have had

rectal polyps	Down's syndrome
rheumatic heart disease	(mongolism)
sickle cell disease	pernicious anemia
syphilis or bad blood	stomach or duodenal ulcer
done [Go to 7]	thyroid disease or goiter
	none of these [Go to 7]

[For each response in the above section, branching to frame 6 will occur. A response on frame 6 will cause return to the frame of the original response.]

6. The person that had this was

my mother	my father
my sister	my brother
one of my grandmothers	one of my grandfathers
an aunt	an uncle
a daughter	a son
	none of these

7. I have blood relatives who have committed suicide (taken their own life).

8. The person that committed suicide was

my mother	my father
my sister	my brother
one of my grandmothers	one of my grandfathers
an aunt	an uncle
a daughter	a son
	none of these

9. My father is still living.

No [Go to 10]   Yes [Go to 11]

10. My father passed away when he was

aged 39 or less   aged 60 to 69
aged 40 to 49   aged 70 or older
aged 50 to 59

11. My mother is still living.

No [Go to 12]   Yes [Go to 13]

12. My mother passed away when she was

aged 39 or less   aged 60 to 69
aged 40 to 49   aged 70 or older
aged 50 to 59

13. My father's father (my paternal grandfather) is still living.

No [Go to 14]   Yes [Go to 15]

14. He passed away when he was

aged 39 or less   aged 60 to 69
aged 40 to 49   aged 70 or older
aged 50 to 59

15. My father's mother (my paternal grandmother) is still living.

No [Go to 16]   Yes [Go to 17]

16. She passed away when she was

aged 39 or less   aged 60 to 69
aged 40 to 49   aged 70 or older
aged 50 to 59

17. My mother's father (my maternal grandfather) is still living.

No [Go to 18]   Yes [Go to 19]

18. He passed away when he was

aged 39 or less   aged 60 to 69
aged 40 to 49   aged 70 or older
aged 50 to 59

19. My mother's mother (my maternal grandmother) is still living.

No [Go to 20]   Yes [Go to next section]

20. She passed away when she was

aged 39 or less   aged 60 to 69
aged 40 to 49   aged 70 or older
aged 50 to 59

INFECTIOUS DISEASE

1. I have had

chicken pox   diphtheria
done   none of these

2. I have had

gonorrhea (or the clap)   malaria
regular measles   German measles
done   none of these

3. I have had hepatitis (yellow jaundice).

4. I have had

mumps   mononucleosis
polio   scarlet fever
done   none of these

5. I have had rheumatic fever.

6. I have had

shingles   spinal meningitis
strep throat   syphilis (or bad blood)
typhoid   tuberculosis (TB)
any tropical disease   whooping cough
done   none of these

IMMUNIZATIONS

1. Within the past 5 years I have had

diphtheria shots   flu shots
gamma globulin shots   none of these
done

2. Within the past 5 years I have had

DPT shots (combined tet-   smallpox vaccination
anus, diphtheria, and   typhoid shots
whooping cough)   none of these
done

3. Within the past 10 years I have had

polio shots   none of these
all 3 oral polio vaccines   done
a tetanus shot

EYE, EAR, NOSE, AND THROAT*

Significance of Response

1. I have had trouble with my eyes.

   past problem

2. I have trouble seeing in the distance or up close.

   refractive error, any cause of ↓ V.A.

3. I have worn or am wearing glasses.

   refractive error or asthenopia

4. Without glasses I can't see in the distance.

   myopia (or older hyperopia) cataracts

5. Without glasses I can't see up close.

   hyperopia or presbyopia

6. I need my glasses for both distance and near.

   high refractive error, astigmatism

7. My vision in one or both eyes is bad without glasses.

   cataract, refractive error, etc.

8. The bad eye is my
   right eye
   left eye
   both eyes

---

* Eye questions documented by Bruce Spivey, M.D., University of Iowa. Ear, nose, and throat questions documented by Loring W. Pratt, M.D., Waterville, Maine.

Significance of Response

9. I have a lazy or wandering   strabismus
   eye.

10. The lazy eye is my
    right eye
    left eye
    both eyes

11. My vision in one eye is not   amblyopia
    improvable to normal
    with glasses.

12. This is my
    right eye
    left eye

13. I have strabismus (crossed   history strabismus
    eyes or wall eyes).

14. I use only one eye at all   strabismus with strong preference
    times.

15. The eye I use is my

    right eye
    left eye

16. I use both eyes but not at   alternating strabismus
    the same time.

17. I see double or used to see   paretic strabismus or intermittent
    double.   deviation

18. I have trouble judging dis-   refractive error or undiagnosed
    tances.   strabismus or nothing

19. I have trouble with   refractive error or undiagnosed
    depth perception.   strabismus or nothing

20. My vision blurs or changes   hyperopia (refractive), strabismus,
    frequently.   glaucoma or diabetes, etc., cata-
                                  racts

21. The blurring is when I   hyperopia (refractive)
    change from near to far
    vision (or vice-versa)

150 · MEDICAL RECORDS, MEDICAL EDUCATION, AND PATIENT CARE

Significance of Response

22. The blurring is mainly in my

    right eye
    left eye
    both eyes

    vascular occlusion?
    (carotid insufficiency)

23. The blurring occurs when I read.

    (hyperopia) refractive or convergence insufficiency

24. The blurring occurs when I am active or shortly after.

    vascular

25. The blurring only comes when I have read for some minutes.

    convergence insufficiency or hyperopia

26. The blurring occurs when I am in a very bright light (especially sunlight).

    cataract

27. The blurring occurs in dim light (e.g., dusk).

    angle closure glaucoma

28. The blurring occurs and lasts nearly all day.

    diabetes or glaucoma

29. I have had several changes of glasses and nothing helps.

    cataract or glaucoma

30. My eyes pain and get red when the vision blurs.

    glaucoma (angle closure)

31. I see spots in front of one eye or both eyes.

    vitreous detachment or degeneration, retinal detachment, uveitis

32. I see spots in front of my

    right eye
    left eye
    both eyes

Significance of Response

33. They are there most of the time, especially when I look at the sky or a blank light wall.

vitreous floaters

34. They appeared suddenly but haven't changed much and I can watch them float away from my sight.

vitreous degeneration

35. The spots look something like cobwebs or a piece of lint.

vitreous degeneration floaters

36. The spots came suddenly, looked like a million red dots and have slowly disappeared.

vitreous hemorrhage, (diabetes, retinal detachment, etc.)

37. The spots were associated with light flashes.

vitreous hemorrhage, probably retinal detachment

38. This happens with my
    right eye
    left eye
    both eyes

39. After the spots a veil slowly came over my eye.

retinal detachment or large vitreous hemorrhages

40. This happened with my
    right eye
    left eye
    both eyes

41. The veil came from:
    right side
    left side
    above
    below

retinal detachment

Significance of Response

42. The spots have slowly
    cleared.

resolving vitreous
hemorrhage or uveitis

43. The spots were worse in
    one part of my vision.

uveitis (localizing)

44. The spots were worse in my
    right eye
    left eye
    they were the same in
       both eyes

45. The spots were worse when I
    looked to the right
    looked to the left
    looked up
    looked down
    done
    none of these

46. My vision is distorted
    centrally.

inflammation in macula,
macular degeneration,
central serous retinopathy

47. The eye that is affected is my
    right eye
    left eye
    both eyes

48. If I look to the side of some-
    thing I see it clearer.

inflammation in macula,
macular degeneration,
central serous retinopathy

49. It has always been this way.
    [If yes, skip to 52]

congenital (example, toxo)

50. It came suddenly.

central serous or hemorrhages
in senile macular degeneration

51. It has gradually appeared.

"senile" macular degeneration

52. I have had an eye operation.

surgery: example, strabismus,
glaucoma, cataracts, retinal
detachment

Significance of Response

53. It was on my

     right eye
     left eye
     both eyes

54. I have had a retinal detachment.

55. It happened in my

     right eye
     left eye
     both eyes

56. I have glaucoma.

57. I have glaucoma in my

     right eye
     left eye
     both eyes

58. I have cataracts.

59. I have them in my

     right eye
     left eye
     both eyes

60. I have uveitis (an inflammation inside my eye).

61. I have had an eye injury requiring surgery.

62. My eyes tear frequently.   nasolacrimal obstruction, inflammation, normal

63. The tears sometimes stream down my face when I am not crying.   causes for epiphora or inflammation

64. This occurs especially when I am outside or in the wind.   normal or nasolacrimal obstruction

Significance of Response

65. The tearing is in my

   right eye
   left eye
   both eyes

66. The tearing has had much   infection or nasolacrimal obstruc-
   mucus or pus associated   tion with dacryocystitis
   with it.

67. Mucus comes from my eye   dacryostenosis with
   when I press near my nose.   dacryocystitis

68. This happens with my

   right eye
   left eye
   both eyes

69. This started after an   dacryocystitis
   infection.

70. This started after an injury.   facial fracture

71. This has been this way all   congenital absence puncta or
   my life.   nasolacrimal obstruction

72. I have had my tear ducts probed.

73. My eye(s) are red frequently.   congenital, hereditary, sleep loss,
   asthenopia, inflammation, blepha-
   ritis, infection, corneal disease

74. This is usually my
   right eye
   left eye
   both eyes

75. This is irritating but has   insignificant blepharitis
   never been a severe
   problem

76. This comes and goes (or is   blepharitis
   worse sometimes than
   others).

Significance of Response

77. I have had treatment but it has never completely disappeared.   blepharitis

78. I have been treated with eyedrops (antibiotics) for this.   blepharitis, virus, etc.

79. I have now or have had an eye infection.   inflammation, uveitis, iritis, corneal conjunctivitis

80. I have had a corneal ulcer.

81. I have this ulcer on my

right eye
left eye
both eyes

82. I was told this infection was a

bacteria
virus
unknown cause

83. I had it once but never again.
[If yes, skip to 87]

84. It has been a recurring problem.   herpes conjunctivitis

85. It happens about

every month
every few months
2 or 3 times a year
once a year
once every few years

86. This has happened a total of

5 times or less
6 to 10 times
11 to 20 times
21 or more times

Significance of Response

87. I have had a cold sore of the eye (herpes).

herpes

88. I have had this sore mainly in my

    right eye
    left eye
    both eyes

89. I have had this cold sore

    1 time
    2 times
    3 times
    4 times
    5 times
    6 times
    7 or more times

90. I have had pink eye but no trouble resulted.

91. I have a scar from an eye infection.

herpes, lues, etc.

92. I am color-blind.

93. I have always been hard of hearing.

congenital or early childhood disease

    No [Go to 94]
    Yes [Go to 97]

94. I have had an infection or injury of my ears or have had a loss of hearing.

    No [Go to 95]
    Yes [Go to 96]

95. People tell me that my hearing is changing.

96. I have had loss of hearing that has not improved very much.

Significance of Response

97. My hearing is getting worse. recent disease

98. I have trouble understand- presbycuesis
    ing the words even if I
    can hear the voice.

99. I have had drainage from otitis media
    an infection in my ear.

100. This has occurred

     only in childhood childhood acute otitis media
     [Go to 104]
     since childhood childhood acute otitis media or
     [Go to 101] long standing chronic otitis media
     only recently recent otitis media
     [Go to 101]

101. It occurs

     off and on probably not mastoid
     continually more like chronic mastoiditis

102. The drainage has a ? bone necrosis; gram-negative
     bad odor. infection

103. At times the discharge is more likely chronic mastoid
     bloody. with cholesteatoma

104. I have had a bad injury to
     my ears.

105. I have had mastoid trouble. history of known disease

106. I often have pain in my ears. temperomandibular joint
     syndrome if no T & A

107. I often have buzzing or tinnitus
     ringing in my ears.

108. I have this buzzing

     all of the time major problem
     when it is quiet minor problem
     when my hearing changes ? Ménière's disease

109. It has occurred only recently. recent change in inner ear

Significance of Response

110. When this buzzing or ring-
 ing happens, I feel dizzy
(as if I'm spinning
around).

? Ménière's disease

111. There is a lot of loud noise
where I work.

history of acoustic trauma

112. I have shot a gun a lot.

history of acoustic trauma

113. In the past, I have had a
serious head injury.

history of head injury

114. At the time of the injury I
lost consciousness (was
knocked out).

severe head injury

115. I bled from my ears with
that injury.

? temporal bone fracture

116. I have been troubled with
nasal discharge (nose drip),
stuffiness, bleeding, and inability to smell things or
have had an injury to my
nose.

117. In the past year I have had
a stuffy nose for a long
period of time.

nasal obstruction

118. This stuffiness happens

only at certain seasons
of the year

allergy

only with colds

upper respiratory infection

all of the time

allergy, foreign body, polyps,
chronic sinusitis

119. The discharge is

clear

allergy

yellow

infection

bloody

? malignancy

Significance of Response

120. I have had nose bleeds not caused by an injury or a cold.

? malignancy

121. I cannot smell things as well as I could, even when I don't have a cold.

122. I have had a serious injury to my nose in the past

? deflected septum

123. A doctor has said that I have polyps in my nose.

124. I have had polyps taken out of my nose.

history of operation

125. I have hard lumps in my tongue or lips.

? tongue or lip lesion

126. The lumps are in

my tongue — ? carcinoma
my lips — ? carcinoma
both my tongue and lips

127. I have noticed sores or spots in my mouth or on my tongue.

128. I have frequent sore throats, even when I don't have a cold.

chronic tonsillitis

129. I have had continual sore throat for a long time— more than 2 weeks.

? carcinoma of pharynx; pyriform sinus or cervical esophagus

130. The pain in my throat seems to run into my ears.

superior laryngeal nerve irritation

131. I have been hoarse for a long time.

? carcinoma of larynx

	Significance of Response
132. I have trouble swallowing food or drink or saliva.	? carcinoma
133. I have trouble swallowing	
solid food	? carcinoma
liquids	? carcinoma-pharyngeal polyp
saliva	? carcinoma-pharyngeal polyp
done	
134. I have had to chew my food more carefully recently.	? carcinoma of esophagus
135. This is getting worse all the time.	carcinoma of esophagus
136. I have coughed up or vomited blood.	? carcinoma
137. I have had food stick in my throat.	stricture
138. I feel like I have a lump in my throat.	globus hystericus if 133, 136, and 137 are negative
139. It is	
recent [Go to 141]	? malignancy
old [Go to 140]	chronic lymphadenitis
140. Has been there since birth.	? congenital cyst (thyroglossal-branchiogenic)
141. My salivary glands swell at times.	chronic sialadenitis
142. This is	
related to eating	calculus
unrelated to eating	? Sjögren's disease
143. I have pain in the joints of my jaws.	temperomandibular joint syndrome
144. My jaw slips out of joint at times.	temperomandibular joint syndrome

Significance of Response

145. My jaw creaks at times.   temperomandibular joint
                               syndrome

146. I have had operations on my
     throat, my nose, or ears.

147. I have had

     my tonsils out   history of operation
     operation on my larynx   history of operation
        (voice box)
     cosmetic surgery on my   history of operation
        nose (had my nose fixed)
     other surgery on my nose   submucous resection; polypectomy
                                        or sinus operation
     none of these
     done

148. I have had

     my ears opened   history of operation
     mastoid surgery   history of operation
     surgery for deafness   history of operation
     tubes put in my ears   history of operation
     done
     none of these

DERMATOLOGY-ALLERGY

1. In the past year I have had problems with my skin or my skin has
   been abnormal (even in just a few places).

2. I had   a red rash   bad itching of the skin   both   neither

3. I had   boils   pimples   both   neither

4. I had   painful open sores   eczema   both   neither

5. I had   hives   psoriasis   both   neither

6. I had   hard lumps in or just under my skin
           infection at the base of a fingernail   both   neither

7. The problems I just talked about started on my
     hands and arms   body (torso)
     feet and legs   face and neck

8. I treated these problems by

> applying something but it
>   didn't help
> applying something and it
>   helped
> I didn't treat them

9. I have noticed

> new growths   sores that won't heal
> moles that are larger   none of the above
>   done

10. I have noticed sores in my
    private regions.

11. I am allergic to some foods.

12. I have an allergy that
    troubles me.

13. When I have this allergy I get

> a rash   hives
> pains or swelling in my   fever
>   joints   none of these things
> difficulty in breathing

14. I have had a bad reaction to a medicine or a shot.

15. I wear a medical identification tag that says that I am allergic to a
certain type of medicine.

16. I know that I am allergic to some medicine or shots or the drink or
pills they give for X ray exams.

17. I am allergic to   penicillin   sulfa drugs   both   neither

18. I am allergic to other antibiotics.

19. I am allergic to aspirin, Empirin, Anacin, or Bufferin.

20. I am allergic to   codeine   morphine   both   neither

21. I am allergic to   Demerol   cortisone-type medicine   both
    neither

22. I am allergic to   phenobarbital   barbituates   both   neither

23. I am allergic to   procaine   Novocaine   both   neither

24. I am allergic to   serum   antitoxin   both   neither

25. I am allergic to drink or pills they give for X ray exams.

26. I am sensitive to detergents, soaps, or shampoos.

27. I am sensitive to cosmetics, hair dyes, or permanent waves.

28. I have often worked around
    chemicals, solvents, or cleaning fluids
    insect or plant sprays
    ammonia, chlorine, or nitrous gases
    engine exhaust fumes (more than 2 hours per day)
    done
    none of the above

29. I have often worked around
    a stone quarry
    plastics or resin fumes
    lead or metal fumes
    asbestos, cement, or
      grain dust
    done

    a coal mine
    X rays or radioactivity
    extreme heat
    coal or granite dust
    none of the above

DENTAL

1. I have been treated by a dentist in the past year.

2. I have had prolonged bleeding when a tooth was pulled.

3. I have been dizzy or have fainted when having dental treatment.

4. I have had a reaction to Novocaine or another dental anesthetic.

5. I have noticed that my gums bleed after I brush my teeth or eat.

6. My teeth feel loose.

7. I have had dental X rays.

8. I sometimes get sores in my mouth.

9. My teeth hurt or ache.

10. The teeth that hurt are
    my top teeth
    my bottom teeth
    both my top and bottom teeth

11. The side of my mouth that hurts most is

my right side
my left side
both sides

12. They hurt most

when I chew
with heat
with cold
without any reason

13. I have a bad taste coming from my teeth or gums.

14. I eat sweets like candy or desserts more than twice a day.

15. I drink pop or soft drinks several times a week.

16. I eat a lot of bread, potatoes, or macaroni.

17. I sometimes eat raw vegetables.

18. I brush my teeth with a toothbrush.

19. I brush my teeth usually about

a few times a week   twice a day
once a day   three times a day

20. I have a history of rheumatism as a child, rheumatic fever, or heart disease.

21. I take fluoride at home for my teeth.

22. I see a dentist regularly to have my teeth checked.

23. I last saw a dentist

within past 6 months   2 to 5 years ago
6 months to 1 year ago   more than 5 years ago
1 to 2 years ago

GASTROINTESTINAL*

Significance of Response

1. I often have a sore tongue.   vitamin B complex deficiencies
(other than B_1) and iron lack

---

* Documentation of gastrointestinal questions by James Butt, M.D., Cleveland Metropolitan General Hospital.

Significance of Response

2. I often have burning or soreness in my mouth and lips.

same as 1 and B$_1$ deficiency

3. I often have sores in my mouth, on my tongue and lips.

aphthous stomatitis (canker sores), herpetic stomatitis, Vincent's stomatitis, leukemia

4. I often have bleeding gums.

pregnancy, chronic gingivitis, aphthous stomatitis, herpetic stomatitis, Vincent's stomatitis, leukemia

5. I often have a feeling of choking or lump in my throat.

6. It occurs

with eating

upper esophageal web (female)

after eating

Zenker's diverticula (male)

not related to eating

depression; hysteria

7. I have trouble swallowing solid foods.

8. It occurs

a. when I first swallow

streptococcal sore throat, tonsillitis, stomatitis, carcinoma of larynx, Plummer-Vinson (Patterson-Kelly syndrome), depression, hysteria, cervical osteophytes

b. after I have begun to swallow

esophagitis, sclerodema, ring, achalasia, diffuse spasm, stricture, tumor, hiatus hernia

9. I have trouble swallowing liquids.

10. It occurs

when I first swallow

same as 8a; more advanced disease

after I have begun to swallow

same as 8b except rings; more advanced disease

11. I have pain on swallowing.

Significance of Response

12. It occurs

    with eating — esophagitis, hiatus hernia, rings, webs, stricture, diffuse spasm, peptic ulcer of esophagus

    after eating — esophagitis, hiatus hernia

    not related to eating — tumor, diffuse spasm

13. It occurs

    when I first swallow — same as 8a; more advanced disease

    after I have begun to swallow — same as 8b; except scleroderma and tumor; more advanced disease

14. The pain frequently radiates into my back — peptic ulcer of esophagus, esophagitis

    into my arms — esophagitis, hiatus hernia

    into my groin and legs — not esophageal pain

    into my chest — peptic ulcer of esophagus, esophagitis

    into my stomach — hiatus hernia, peptic ulcer of esophagus

    it doesn't radiate at all

15. It is

    burning in nature — esophagitis; scleroderma

    sticking in nature — achalasia, webs, ring, stricture

    intense — esophagitis, hiatus hernia, peptic ulcer of esophagus, achalasia,

    aching in nature — tumor, hernia

    cramping in nature

    gnawing in nature

    none of these

16. It is relieved by

    sitting, standing up, or stretching — hiatus hernia, esophagitis, achalasia, ring, stricture

	Significance of Response
antacids (such as Tums, soda, Maalox, Alka-Seltzer)	esophagitis, peptic ulcer of esophagus
bending over or having a bowel movement	achalasia, ring, stricture
nothing	tumor, peptic ulcer of esophagus, diffuse spasm
food	esophagitis
milk	esophagitis, peptic ulcer of esophagus
vomiting	hiatus hernia, achalasia, diffuse spasm
something not listed	

17. It is aggravated by

lying down	hernia, esophagitis, peptic ulcer of esophagus
food	esophagitis, peptic ulcer of esophagus, achalasia, ring, stricture, tumor
especially fatty foods	esophagitis, hernia, peptic ulcer of esophagus
bending over	esophagitis, hiatus hernia, peptic ulcer of esophagus
aspirin	esophagitis, hiatus hernia
something not listed	

18. This pain occurs

every day or nearly every day	tumor, web, stricture, ring, achalasia, peptic ulcer of esophagus, esophagitis
several times a week	esophagitis, hiatus hernia, diffuse spasm
a few times a month	diffuse spasm, hiatus hernia
a few times a year	hiatus hernia

Significance of Response

19. The pain usually starts

    when I am hungry — esophagitis, peptic ulcer of esophagus

    right after I have eaten — esophagitis, hiatus hernia

    an hour or two after eating — esophagitis, peptic ulcer of esophagus

    in the middle of the night, waking me up — esophagitis, hiatus hernia

20. I have had X rays taken of my esophagus (the tube from my mouth to my stomach).

21. I recently have been troubled by a poor appetite. — hepatitis; cirrhosis; tumor

22. In the past year I have gained or lost more than ten pounds without trying to.

23. I have gained ten pounds or more. — congestive heart failure, renal disease, recovery from illness, growth, overeating due to depression or anxiety

24. I have lost ten pounds or more. — evidence of systemic disease

25. I often have pain in my stomach.

26. It occurs

    with eating — peptic ulcer, carcinoma, irritable colon, mesenteric vascular insufficiency

	Significance of Response
after eating	peptic ulcer, carcinoma, biliary-pancreatic disease, ulcerative colitis, Crohn's diseases, irritable colon
not related to eating	penetrating ulcer, Crohn's diseases, ulcerative colitis, functional GI disorder

27. It is

burning in nature	gastritis
sticking in nature	Crohn's diseases of bowel; functional GI disorder
intense	peptic ulcer, peritoneal pain, irritable colon, ulcerative colitis, Crohn's diseases of bowel, mesenteric vascular insufficiency, pancreatitis, tumor, biliary tract disease
aching in nature	peptic ulcer, cholecystitis, Crohn's diseases, cholelithiasis, tumor
cramping in nature	colic (biliary, colonic renal, mesenteric vascular insufficiency)
gnawing in nature	peptic ulcer, cancer of stomach
none of these	

28. The pain frequently radiates

into my back	penetrating ulcer, perforation into lesser sac, pancreatitis, tumor, biliary tract diseases
into my arms	gastritis
into my groin and legs	
into my chest	biliary tract
into my stomach	peritoneal, appendicitis, biliary-pancreatic tract
it doesn't radiate at all	

Significance of Response

29. It is usually located

above my navel	duodenal, liver, biliary and pancreatic tracts
below my navel	appendicitis, distal ileum and caecum, right and left colon
above and below my navel	peritoneum, vascular insufficiency
at the level of my navel	distal duodenum, jejuno-ileum, right colon, left colon

30. It usually occurs on

the right side of my stomach	duodenum, liver, biliary-pancreatic tract, ileum, right colon and appendix peritoneum
on the left side of my stomach	pancreatic tract, lesser peritoneal sac, left colon
both sides of my stomach	right and left colon, peritoneum
in the middle of my stomach	distal duodenum, jejuno-ileum, mesenteric vasculature; peritoneum

31. This pain occurs

every day or nearly every day	peptic ulcer, tumor, colitis, enteritis
several times a week	peptic ulcer, tumor
a few times a month	biliary-pancreatic tract disease, peptic ulcer
a few times a year	biliary-pancreatic tract disease, peptic ulcer

32. This pain usually starts

when I am hungry	peptic ulcer, tumor
right after I have eaten	peptic ulcer, tumor, Crohn's diseases of bowel, ulcerative colitis, biliary-pancreatic tract

Significance of Response

an hour or two after eating peptic ulcer, tumor, biliary-pancreatic tract disease

in the middle of the night, waking me up peptic ulcer, tumor

none of these

33. It is relieved by

sitting, standing up, or stretching pancreatic or hepatic disease

antacids, (such as Tums, soda, Maalox, Alka-Seltzer) peptic ulcer, tumor

bending over or having a bowel movement colitis, pancreatic disease, Crohn's diseases of bowel

nothing tumor, penetrating ulcer, colitis, Crohn's diseases of bowel

food peptic ulcer, gastric ca, gastritis

milk peptic ulcer, gastric ca

vomiting peptic ulcer, gastric ca, gastritis

something not listed

34. It is aggravated by

lying down pancreatic disease

food peptic ulcer, pancreatic disease, Crohn's diseases of bowel, ulcerative colitis

especially fatty foods gastritis; biliary tract disorders

bending over peritoneal disease

aspirin peptic ulcer, tumor

something not listed

35. I have recently been troubled with nausea or vomiting. peptic ulcer, tumor, hepatobiliary, pancreatic tract disease

36. In the past I have vomited blood, or brown- or coffee-ground-colored material. peptic ulcer, tumor, varices, gastritis, esophagitis

Significance of Response

37. I have had X rays taken of my stomach (X rays taken of stomach area after drinking chalk-like liquid).

38. I have been told that I have ulcers in my stomach or intestine.

39. The ulcers are in

    my stomach
    my intestine
    both stomach and intestine

40. I have had an operation on my stomach.

41. I have had liver disease.

42. I have had jaundice (have had yellow skin or yellow eyes).

43. I have been told that I had gall bladder trouble.

44. I have had X rays taken of my gall bladder (X rays taken of stomach area after taking many large white pills the night before).

45. I have been told that I had gall stones.

46. I have had an operation on my gall bladder.

47. It was removed.

Significance of Response

48. I have had X rays taken of my intestine (X rays taken of stomach area after being given a barium enema in which fluid was pumped up my rectum).

49. I have had an operation on my intestines.

50. The operation was on my

    large intestine
    small intestine
    both large and small
    intestines

51. I have had my appendix taken out.

52. I have frequent loose stools, more than 3 times daily. — colitis, irritable colon, malabsorption, anxiety state, hyperthyroidism

53. I often have cramping and gas with my bowel movements. — colitis, irritable colon, malabsorption, anxiety state, hyperthyroidism

54. I have recently had to get up in the middle of the night to have a bowel movement. — serious diarrheal problem requiring investigation

55. I sometimes have trouble controlling my bowels. — serious diarrheal problem, colitis, malabsorption, anxiety state

56. My stools are often mixed with mucus or slime. — anxiety state

57. I have much less frequent bowel movements than before. — depression; anxiety state, early obstructive symptoms, either anatomic (tumor) or functional (colitis)

Significance of Response

58. I use more laxatives than I used to.

anxiety state or depression

59. My stools frequently are smaller than they used to be.

cancer of rectum; fissure; proctitis; anxiety state

60. My stools are thin and narrow, like a pencil.

cancer of rectum; fissure; proctitis, anxiety state

61. I often have black, tarry stools.

serious GI bleeding, i.e., requiring investigation

62. This occurs only when I take iron medicine, Pepto Bismol, or vitamins.

63. My stools are mixed with blood.

serious GI bleeding, i.e., requiring investigation—bleeding above rectum

64. My stools are frequently covered with blood.

serious GI bleeding, i.e., requiring investigation, commonly hemorrhoids, rectal carcinoma

65. My stools are often extremely foul and smelly.

suspicious but far from diagnostic for steatorrhea, anxiety state

66. My stools often float on top of the water.

suspicious but not alone diagnostic for steatorrhea

67. My stools are often fluffy, greasy, or frothy

same as 66

68. They often leave the toilet greasy.

same as 66

69. My stools are very bulky.

same as 66

70. I often use laxatives.

obsessive personality; alkalosis, hypochloremic may have smooth left colon on barium enema resembling ulcerative colitis

71. I often take an enema.   same as 70

72. I have been told that I had
    colon or bowel disease.

73. I have been told that I had
    dysentery.

74. I have been told that I had
    worms.

75. I have been told that I had
    hemorrhoids (piles).

76. I have been bothered by
    hemorrhoids recently.

77. I have had recent trouble
    with my rectum (hemor-
    rhoids don't count).

78. I have an anal fissure.

79. I have a pain in my rectum.

80. I have an itching or burning
    of my rectum.

81. My bowel wall seems to come   chronic diarrheal states
    out with my bowel
    movements.

82. I have had a serious injury   pancreatitis, ruptured viscus, ob-
    to my stomach or stomach   structive hematoma, infarction
    organs.   of bowel

83. I am concerned that I might
    have serious stomach or
    intestinal trouble now.

HEMATOPOIETIC

1. When I cut myself, I bleed more than I think is normal.

2. I have been told that I am a hemophiliac or a bleeder.

3. There is someone in my family who is a hemophiliac.

4. I sometimes get black and blue spots for no reason.

5. I have been told that I am anemic or have low blood.

6. I had a blood test done when I was told I was anemic.

7. I have taken anemia or iron medicine in the past year.

8. I am taking this medicine now.

9. I have taken other medicine for my blood.

10. I have been told that I have or have had

sickle cell disease	polycythemia
pernicious anemia	done
leukemia	none of these
infectious mononucleosis	

11. In the past year I have had enlarged glands or lumps in my armpits, groin or neck.

12. I have had enlarged glands or lumps in my neck in the past year.

13. I have had enlarged glands or lumps in my armpits in the past year.

14. I have had enlarged glands or lumps in my groin in the past year.

15. I have had a blood transfusion in the past.

16. I had a transfusion reaction when I had a transfusion.

17. I have recurring fevers.

18. A doctor has told me that I had too many or too few white blood cells or red blood cells.

19. He said that I had too many white blood cells.

20. He said that I had too few white blood cells.

21. He said that I had too many red blood cells.

22. I have given blood.

23. I have tried to give blood but the blood was rejected.

24. I have had large amounts of blood drawn because of a disease (phlebotomy).

25. I have other problems with my blood that I know about, or I am afraid I might have other problems with my blood.

RESPIRATORY*

Significance of Response

1. I have a cough (even a cigarette cough counts).

   acute or chronic infection, chronic bronchitis, bronchial tumor, pulmonary embolus, broncholith, bronchiectasis

2. This cough started about

   within the past 24 hours — acute situation
   a day to a week ago
   a week to a month ago — becoming chronic
   1 month to 6 months ago
   6 months to 12 months ago
   1 to 2 years ago
   2 to 3 years ago — 2 years chronic bronchitis a major consideration
   3 to 5 years ago
   6 or more years ago

3. This cough has

   gotten worse since starting
   stayed the same since starting
   improved since starting

   } suggests the pattern of the illness: progressive, stable, regressive

---

* Documentation of respiratory questions by Gerald L. Baum, M.D., Veterans Administration Hospital, Cleveland, and by D. G. Gilespie, M.D., Cleveland Metropolitan General Hospital.

Significance of Response

4. This cough starts

   in my throat
   in my neck
   in the bronchial tubes
   deep in my chest
   I'm not sure where it starts

   } suggests bronchi or pulmonary parenchyma as the source

5. It starts

   as soon as I sit up
   after a cup of coffee or
      hot liquid
   after my first cigarette
   not until I go outside
   none of these

   } implies the cough is in response to secretions that were present in tracheobronchial tree for an hour or more

6. I usually cough first thing in the morning.

   chronic bronchitis, emphysema, smoker, chronic sinusitis

7. I cough quite a lot (several times) during the day.

   active and/or persistent underlying process

8. I cough at night

   more than during the day
   less than during the day

   } this indicates that gravity worsens cough or not, when patient is in horizontal position, suggesting pooled secretions

9. The cough sometimes wakes me up during the night.

10. The cough keeps me awake during the night and I can't go to sleep.

11. The cough is relieved if I sit up or use more than one pillow.

12. I cough several months out of the year.

    chronic bronchitis or bronchiectasis

Significance of Response

13. I have chest pain when I cough.

association of cough and pain suggests infection. If pain pleuritic in character, pneumonia and/or abscess may be present. Raw mid-localized pain characteristic of acute bronchitis.

14. The pain is mainly in my

    right side
    left side
    front middle
    back middle
    none of these

15. It is

    sharp
    dull
    raw
    none of these
    done

16. I bring up phlegm (sputum, mucus) from my chest when I cough.

17. I bring up

    more than ¼ cup per day
    less than ¼ cup per day

    quantity and character of sputum indicate infectious nature of process or suggest chronic bronchitis or abscess

18. The phlegm (sputum, mucus) is

    clear
    yellow or green
    none of these

19. This happens mostly early in the morning.

20. It smells and/or tastes bad.

Significance of Response

21. I have coughed up phlegm for
   one day only
   up to one week
   up to one month
   up to 6 months
   up to a year   } chronic bronchitis and emphysema
   up to 4 years
   5 years or more

22. The amount of phlegm has
   increased since this
      started
   decreased since this   } implies progression, stability, or regression of process
      started
   remained the same
   increased   bronchiectasis,
                             chronic bronchitis

23. I have coughed up blood.

24. This has happened

                             bronchiectasis, tumor and/or tuberculosis if > 40; acute pneumonia broncholith if < 40; infarct. abscess at any age. [Also applies to questions 25 and 26]
   only with current illness
   before current illness

25. Now I cough up blood
   rarely
   frequently

26. When I cough up blood it is a
   streaking of sputum only
   large amount of blood in
      phlegm

27. I am sometimes short of   ventilatory impairment, get
   breath or am short of   pulmonary function
   breath now.

Significance of Response

28. I get short of breath when I exercise (heavy work, going up 25 stairs, running).   must differentiate between cardiac and pulmonary cause of dyspnea

29. I get short of breath walking up 15 stairs or on level ground after 180 feet.

30. I often get short of breath just sitting still.

31. There are times when I just can't seem to get enough air even at rest.   this suggests anxiety

32. I have had shortness of breath with wheezing.   this implies a spastic or reversible bronchial obstruction

33. My shortness of breath problem started about

    within the past 24 hours } pulmonary embolus, pneumotho-
    a day to a week ago   } rax, pneumonia

    a week to a month ago
    1 month to 6 months ago
    6 months to 12 months ago } chronic obstructive
    1 to 2 years ago   } lung disease
    2 to 3 years ago
    3 to 5 years ago
    6 or more years ago

34. This shortness of breath problem is

    staying about the same } the pattern suggests a progressive
    getting better   } or stable process

    varies day to day
    getting worse slowly   } bronchitis, pulmonary emphy-
    getting worse rapidly   } sema; asthma is suggested by epi-
    (spells of severe short- } sodic nature
    ness of breath)

35. I have been told that I have emphysema.

Significance of Response

36. I have had blood studies done to measure oxygen and carbon dioxide in my blood (blood gas studies).

37. I have had blowing (breathing) tests.

38. I have had extreme pain when breathing.

39. It lasted

minutes	character and duration of pain
hours	suggest pleura, heart or upper gas-
days	trointestinal tract as site of
weeks	pathology

40. It is helped by pressure over the chest.

41. It was associated with a raspy sensation.

42. It comes and goes.

43. I have had water removed from my lungs or chest.

44. This happened

only with my present illness	pleurisy with effusion associated
once or twice before	with pneumonia, cardiac failure,
many times before	or tuberculosis

45. I get short of breath when the water comes.

46. I have had a collapsed lung.

47. This has happened

| only once | bullous disease > 40 years of age, |
| several times | ruptured pleural blebs < 30 years of age |

Significance of Response

48. It was collapsed by a doctor.   tuberculosis

49. I have fever now.   infection and/or tumor

50. I know this
    by thermometer
    only by my feel

51. I have had fever in the past
    only occasionally with bad ⎫   recurrent febrile episodes suggest
        colds, the flu, etc.   ⎬   bronchiectasis or abscess. If several
    on and off without ap- ⎬   in 1–2 years, suggest pneumonia
        parent acute infections ⎭   behind an obstructing tumor

52. I sometimes sweat so much   suggest chronic debility
    during the night that the
    bedclothes get wet.

53. I have lost weight (more than
    10 pounds).

54. I have lost weight
    only with acute present   weight loss over 10 lbs. implies
        illness   tumor or progressive granuloma-
    over many months   tous disease
    over more than one year

55. I have had
    bronchitis   hay fever
    emphysema   sinus trouble
    pneumonia   none of these
    done

56. I have recently had asthma.

57. I had asthma as a child.

58. I have had pulmonary
    tuberculosis (TB).

59. I have had contact with a
    person with tuberculosis
    (TB).

60. I have had a positive tuber-   especially helpful if current
    culosis (TB) skin test.   test shows change

Significance of Response

61. I have had a chest X ray
    in the past year.

62. I have had an abnormal
    chest X ray film.

63. I smoke cigarettes now.   smoking with inhaling associated
                                   with bronchogenic tumor and
                                   chronic bronchitis

64. I (now) smoke about
    less than a pack per day
    1 pack per day
    1 to 2 packs per day
    2 or more packs per day
    [Go to 68]

65. I used to smoke cigarettes.

66. I quit in
    last 6 months
    last year
    last 2 years
    last 5 years or more

67. I did smoke about
    less than a pack per day
    1 pack per day
    1 to 2 packs per day
    2 or more packs per day

68. In all I have smoked cigarettes
    less than a year   1 to 2 years
    3 to 5 years   6 to 10 years
    11 to 20 years   21 to 30 years
    31 to 40 years   more than 40 years

69. I smoke cigars.

70. I inhale the cigar smoke.

Significance of Response

71. I smoke a pipe.

72. I inhale the pipe smoke.

73. I have had a period of prolonged hoarseness or have hoarseness now.

bronchogenic ca; laryngeal tumor; tuberculosis

74. In the past I have injured my chest.

may account for skeletal or pleural abnormalities

75. I have had an operation on my chest.

previous tumor, tuberculosis, abscess, bronchiectasis

76. In the past I have had broken ribs.

often associated with alcoholism and tuberculosis

CARDIOVASCULAR*

Significance of Response

1. I have been told that I have heart disease.

2. I have known that I have heart disease since

birth	probably congenital
age 5 to 10	probably rheumatic
age 10 to 20	probably rheumatic
age 20 to 40	probably rheumatic
age 40 to 50	(male) probably hypertensive arteriosclerotic
age 50 or older	probably hypertensive arteriosclerotic

3. Within the past year I have had pain, pressure, or a tight feeling in my chest.

* Documentation of cardiovascular questions by Louis Rakita, M.D., Cleveland Metropolitan General Hospital.

Significance of Response

4. It is

a burning sensation
a sharp pain
a tearing pain
a dull pain
a squeezing pain
can't describe

} useful with other information to differentiate etiology from coronary, esophageal, aortic, or pleural

5. I have had this pain in my chest for

6 months or less
6 months to 1 year
1 to 2 years
2 to 5 years
more than 5 years

} acute or chronic (coronary insufficiency, dissecting aneurysm, etc., and degree of acuteness or chronicity)

6. The pain started

suddenly   acute coronary insuffic.
gradually   chronic coronary insuffic.

7. The current pain started

1 day ago
2 days ago
3 days ago
4 days ago
more than 4 days ago

} useful in interpreting enzyme changes present and thus cause; aggressiveness of therapy if MI present

8. The pain comes from under   coronary
my breastbone (in the
middle of my chest)

9. It comes from

the far left side of my chest
the far right side of my chest
both sides of my chest
none of these

} localization helpful in pinpointing system and etiology, such as pleural, musculoskeletal

Significance of Response

10. The pain stays in one place.   pleural vs coronary vs aortic vs esophageal

11. It radiates (shoots) to
    one arm   coronary
    my abdomen   dissection
    my chin or jaw   coronary or dissection
    my back   coronary or dissection
    some place not listed
    it doesn't radiate or shoot

12. The pain is
    continuous [Go to 13]   coronary, dissection
    intermittent (comes and   gall bladder
    goes) [Go to 18]

13. The pain is made worse   coronary
    when I get annoyed or
    excited.

14. The pain is worse after I eat.   coronary

15. The pain is made worse   coronary
    when I have sexual inter-
    course (sex relations).

16. The pain is made worse   coronary
    when I exercise.

17. The pain is made worse   pleural
    when I cough or breathe.
    [Go to 25]

18. The pain lasts
    more than a minute   transient coronary insuf.
    more than 10 minutes   acute coronary insuf.
       $\bar{s}$ infarction
    more than 30 minutes
    more than 1 hour   myocardial infarction

19. The pain sometimes comes   coronary
    when I am sitting still.

Significance of Response

20. The pain sometimes comes when I get annoyed or excited. coronary

21. The pain sometimes comes after a big meal. coronary

22. The pain sometimes comes when I have sexual inter-course (sex relations). coronary

23. The pain sometimes comes when I exercise. coronary

24. The pain sometimes comes when I cough. pleural

25. It sometimes makes me sick to my stomach. gastrointestinal (gall bladder) vs coronary

26. It sometimes wakes me up in the middle of the night. GI, occasional coronary

27. I take medicine to relieve the pain. coronary, GI

28. The pain is relieved by eating. GI

29. The pain is relieved when I rest. coronary

30. The pain first started after eating something sharp like a chicken bone. trauma

31. This pain keeps me from doing what I would like to do. severity, psychogenic

32. I have to sit up to sleep. heart failure

33. I can feel my heart beat in an unusual way. arrhythmia

34. This beating bothers me. tolerance

	Significance of Response
35. My heart often thumps and races even when I am resting.	arrhythmia
36. The fast beating starts and stops very suddenly.	paroxysmal atrial tachycardia
37. My heart always beats very fast.	hyperthyroidism
38. It sometimes beats very slowly.	heart block
39. My heart occasionally skips a beat or has an extra beat.	premature beats, heart block
40. I have often had painless swelling in my feet or ankles.	heart failure, estrogens, idiopathic
41. This swelling happens in	
one foot or one ankle	local disease
both feet or both ankles	heart failure
42. This swelling goes down overnight.	heart failure
43. [Women] This was worse when I was pregnant.	severity of heart disease
44. I sometimes wake up in the middle of the night with a smothering feeling.	left ventricular failure
45. I have been taking heart medicine.	severity of disease, drug induced arrhythmias, type of disease
46. I have been taking it for	
a few weeks or less	
a few months	duration disease, drug induced
1 to 2 years	arrhythmias, type of disease
2 or more years	

Significance of Response

47. I know the name of my heart medicine.

48. It is
    digitalis   Coumadin
    quinidine   Pronestyl (procainamide)
    nitroglycerine   other name

49. I am on or have been on a salt-free diet.   heart failure

50. I am following it.   }   patient's motivation
    I am not following it. }   severity of disease

51. I have taken high blood pressure medicine.   hypertension

52. I know the name of my high blood pressure medicine.

53. It is
    guanethidine (Ismelin)
    methyldopa (Aldomet)
    thiazides (Diuril, Esi-
        drix, Renese)
    hydralazine (Apresoline)
    reserpine (Serpasil)
    other not listed

54. I am taking anti-coagulant medicine (blood-thinning pills).

55. I have taken shots or pills to lose water.   heart failure

56. I am taking them now.   chronic or acute problem, transient or long standing

57. They cause me to lose
    a little water
    a moderate amount of   }   effectiveness of therapy; will other
        water   approaches be required
    a large amount of water }

Significance of Response

58. I have taken chest pain pills   angina pectoris
     I put under my tongue.

59. I am taking them now.   acute, recent, or chronic

60. They give

     immediate relief
     no relief
     relief in several minutes   } effectiveness of RX and need for further therapy
     partial relief
     relief in several hours

61. I have leg cramps that some-
     times wake me up during
     the night.

62. I have leg pains that some-   periph. vasc. disease
     times make me stop walk-
     ing, and they leave after
     I rest for a while.

63. They come after

     walking one block   } severity,
     walking ½ mile or more   Leriche syndrome
     walking several blocks

64. I have pain in my buttocks   Leriche syndrome
     when I have these leg
     pains.

65. I have varicose veins in my   venous disease
     legs (veins that stick out).

66. My fingers become numb,   Raynaud's disease
     painful, or show unusual
     color when they get cool.

67. The skin on the lower part   vascular disease
     of my legs has become
     darker in color.

Significance of Response

68. The skin on the lower part
    of my legs

        feels thick and tough to   vascular disease
          touch

        is becoming smooth, shiny,   vascular disease
          and hairless

        is all right

69. The skin on the lower part   vascular disease
    of my legs has sores that
    are slow to heal.

70. A doctor told me that I had

        an abnormal electro-
          cardiogram (EKG)   past history of heart
        an abnormal chest X ray   disease
        angina pectoris
        none of these
        done

71. A doctor told me that I had

        a blood clot in an artery   thrombosis or embolism
          (an embolus)

        a blood clot in a vein   thrombosis or embolism
          (phlebitis or thrombo-
          phlebitis)

        an enlarged heart   prior heart disease
        none of these
        done

72. A doctor told me that I had

        a heart attack or coronary
        a heart murmur
        low blood pressure
        scarlet fever   actual or potential
        heart failure   heart disease
        high blood pressure
        rheumatic fever
        none of these
        done

Significance of Response

73. I am worried about my heart, and I have never had a satisfactory explanation.   anxiety

MUSCULOSKELETAL

1. As a child I had trouble with my arms or legs, or I walked with a limp.

2. I have a deformity in my arms or legs.

3. I have had this since
   birth
   childhood
   adulthood

4. This deformity interferes with my daily life.

5. I had difficulty participating in sports when I was young.

6. I had problems with my coordination.

7. I had a hard time doing exercises.

8. I have problems with my coordination now (my arms or legs feel awkward and clumsy).

9. I have had some trouble with my arms, legs, hands, feet, or joints (such as broken bones, strains, painful, infected, or stiff joints, etc.).

10. I have had one or more broken bones in my arms, legs, hands, feet, ankles, knees, or elbows.

11. I broke my
arm	leg
wrist	hand
knee	ankle
elbow	foot
done	bone not listed

12. I have had injuries to my arms, legs, hands, or feet, but they were not broken.

13.   These injuries included

strains	sprains
bad bruises	done

14.   I have had a bone or joint in my arm, leg, hand, or foot operated on.

15.   The operation was on my

arm	leg
wrist	hand
knee	ankle
elbow	foot
done	bone not listed

16. I have had painful joints.

17. This is a problem now.

18. It involves my

hips	shoulders
knees	elbows
ankles	wrists
feet	hands
fingers	toes
done	none of these

19. There is also

swelling	redness
heat	drainage
done	none of these

20. I have had an infected joint.

21.   I have had fluid or pus drawn off with a needle.

22.   I have had medications injected into a joint.

23.   My joints have recently been stiff.

24.   This happens only in the morning.

25.   This is the result of an injury.

26. I have trouble moving around (use crutches, can't get off bus, etc.), or have trouble using my hands to do things.

27.   I have trouble walking.

28.   I need to use crutches, a cane, or a walker regularly.

29.   I use
      a walker   a cane
      one crutch   two canes
      two crutches

30.   I have trouble getting dressed.

31.   I am unable to put on my shoes and socks by myself.

32.   I have trouble buttoning buttons.

33.   I have trouble getting to the bathroom.

34.   [Men] I have trouble shaving.

35.   I have trouble combing my hair.

36.   I have trouble getting up or sitting down.

37.   I have trouble opening a door.

38.   I have trouble holding a glass.

39.   I have trouble getting on or off the bus.

40.   I have trouble getting up or down stairs.

41.   I have to climb more than one flight of stairs to get to where I live.

42.   In the past, I have had trouble with my back (pain, operation, injury, etc.).

43.   I have had back pain that interferes with things I want to do.

44.   The pain is
      low down in my back (hip level)
      middle or high up in my back (chest level)
      shooting down my legs.

45.   I have back pain now.

46.   I have had this back pain for
      more than 6 months   less than 6 months

47.   My back pain is
      getting better
      getting worse
      staying the same

48.   The back pain is worse after I get into bed.

49.   I have injured my back in the past.

50.   I have had my back operated on.

51.   In the past, I have had trouble with my neck (pain, operation, injury, etc.).

52.   I have had neck pain that interferes with things I want to do.

53.   I have this neck pain now.

54.   I have had this neck pain for
      more than 6 months   less than 6 months

55.   This neck pain is
      getting better
      getting worse
      staying the same

56.   I have injured my neck in the past.

57.   In this injury
      I broke my neck   I strained my neck   I had a whiplash injury

58.   I have had my neck operated on.

59.   In the past, I have had trouble with my hip (pain, operation, injury, etc.).

60.   I have had hip pain that interferes with things I want to do.

61.   I have this hip pain now.

62.   I have had this hip pain for
      more than 6 months   less than 6 months

63.   This hip pain is
      getting better
      getting worse
      staying the same

64.   I have injured my hip in the past.

65.   In this injury
      I broke my hip   I strained my hip

66.   I have had my hip operated on.

67.   One of my legs is shorter than the other.

68.   In the past, I have had trouble with my shoulder (pain, operation, injury, etc.).

69.   I have had shoulder pain that interferes with things I want to do.

70.   I have this shoulder pain now.

71. I have had this shoulder pain for
      more than 6 months   less than 6 months

72. This shoulder pain is
      getting better
      getting worse
      staying the same

73. In the past I have injured my shoulder
      not all all [Go to 75]
      one time
      two times   } [Go to 74]
      three or more times

74. In this injury (injuries)
      I broke my shoulder   I strained my shoulder
      I dislocated my shoulder   done

75. I have had my shoulder operated on.

76. I have had a fractured skull.

77. I have had broken ribs.

78. I have been told that I have gout, lupus, or arthritis.

79. I have been told that I have gout.

80. I am presently taking or should be taking gout medicine.

81. I know the name of my gout medicine.

82. It is
      Benemid   Phenylbutazone
      Colchicine   Xyloprim (Allopurinol)
      Cortisone   other not listed

83. I am on a low purine diet.

84. I have been told I have arthritis.

85. I am presently taking or should be taking medicine for my arthritis.

86. The medicine I am taking or should be taking is
      Aspirin or Bufferin   Anacin
      Cortisone   Empirin
      Indocin   Phenacetin
      PAC (APC)   Gold
                      other not listed

87. I have been told I have lupus.

88. I am presently taking or should be taking medicine for my lupus.

89. I have had trouble with my muscles (not because of overexercise), such as swelling, tenderness, weakness, wasting (or shrinking), cramping, or paralysis.

90. I have had muscle swelling within the past 6 months.

91. I have had muscle tenderness within the past 6 months.

92. I have had a paralyzed limb in the past.

93. I have had muscle weakness within the past 6 months.

94. This weakness involves

    all of my muscles   some of my muscles

95. I think that this weakness is due mainly to fatigue (loss of pep, tiredness).

96. Some of my muscles have become shrunken or wasted.

97. This is because of

    previous illness   other reason
    previous injury   I don't know why

98. I am troubled by cramps in the muscles of my legs.

99. They usually occur

    while I am exercising (as in walking)
    after I exercise
    while I am in bed at night

100. My posture has recently been changing.

101. I regularly take aspirin for joint or muscle pains.

102. I have been given rheumatism medicine.

103. I have noticed that I am getting shorter.

ENDOCRINE

1. In the past six months my appetite has
    increased   decreased   stayed about the same

2. I wear more clothes in cold weather than I used to.

3. My hands tremble or shake most of the time.

4. I perspire more than I used to.

5. I have been told that my eyes bulge out more than they used to.

6. A doctor has told me that I had thyroid or goiter trouble, or I have taken thyroid pills or had an operation on my thyroid.

7. A doctor has told me that I have an overactive thyroid gland or excess thyroid.

8. A doctor has told me that I have a goiter.

9. A doctor has told me that I have an underactive thyroid or lack of thyroid.

10. In the past, I have taken thyroid pills.

11. I have had an operation on my thyroid or goiter.

12. Since reaching adult life, I have noticed an increase in the size of my head (hat size) or hands (glove size).

13. Within the past year my weight has

    increased   decreased
    [Go to 14, then 15, then 17] [Go to 14, 15, 16, 17]
    stayed about the same
    [Go to 17]

14. The change has been about

    5 pounds   20 to 30 pounds
    5 to 10 pounds   30 to 40 pounds
    10 to 20 pounds   more than 40 pounds

15. This change happened in about

    less than a month   8 to 12 months
    1 to 2 months   more than a year
    3 to 5 months
    6 to 8 months

16. This loss of weight happened

    for no reason
    because of dieting
    because I have been taking weight-reducing pills
    because I have been taking water pills
    because I have lost my appetite

17. The least I have weighed as an adult was

less than 80 to 90
  pounds
90 to 100 pounds
100 to 110 pounds
110 to 120 pounds
120 to 130 pounds
} [Go to 19]

130 to 140 pounds
140 to 150 pounds
150 to 160 pounds
160 to 170 pounds
more than 170
  pounds
} [Go to 19]

18. The least I have weighed as an adult was

170 to 180 pounds
180 to 190 pounds
190 to 200 pounds
200 to 210 pounds

210 to 220 pounds
220 to 230 pounds
230 to 240 pounds
more than 240 pounds

19. When I weighed this amount I was about

less than 20 years old
20 to 30 years old
30 to 40 years old
40 to 50 years old

50 to 60 years old
60 to 70 years old
70 to 80 years old
more than 80 years old

20. [Women] The most I have weighed as an adult (excluding pregnancy) is
    or
21. [Men] The most I have weighed as an adult is

80 to 90 pounds
90 to 100 pounds
100 to 110 pounds
110 to 120 pounds
120 to 130 pounds
} [Go to 23]

130 to 140 pounds
140 to 150 pounds
150 to 160 pounds
160 to 170 pounds
more than 170
  pounds
} [Go to 23]

22. The most I have weighed as an adult is

170 to 180 pounds
180 to 190 pounds
190 to 200 pounds
200 to 210 pounds

210 to 220 pounds
220 to 230 pounds
230 to 240 pounds
more than 240 pounds

23. This is the amount I weigh now.

Yes [Go to 25]   No [Go to 24]

24. When I weighed this amount I was about

    less than 20 years old   50 to 60 years old
    20 to 30 years old   60 to 70 years old
    30 to 40 years old   70 to 80 years old
    40 to 50 years old   more than 80 years old

25. A doctor has told me that I have diabetes ("sugar").

26. I have taken insulin.

27. I am taking insulin.

28. I have taken diabetes pills.

29. I am taking diabetes pills.

30. I have had sugar in my urine.

31. [Women] I have had sugar in my urine

    when I was pregnant   during and after I was pregnant
    between the times I was   I have never been pregnant
    pregnant

32. I am more thirsty now than I used to be.

33. I have noticed that my mouth is dry and sticky.

34. I crave salt more than I used to.

35. I have lost some or much of the hair around my sex organs, in my armpits, or all over my body.

36. I have lost this hair from

    around my sex organs   my armpits
    my armpits and around   all over my body
    my sex organs

37. The hair on my head is thinner now or coming out in patches.

38. [Women] I find it necessary to shave the hair on my face.

39. [Men] I started shaving when I was between the ages of 13 to 18 years old.

40. [Men] I have been given hormones for prostate trouble.

41. In the past six months I have taken ACTH, cortisone, prednisone, or similar hormones.

42. I have noticed a change in my sex drive or nature.

43. I have noticed a change in the color or texture of my skin.

44. The change has been in
     the color
     the texture
     both color and texture

BREAST
[For use in detecting carcinoma of the breast]

1. I have had lumps, open sores, abscesses, or discharge from my breasts or nipples or an infection of my nipples.

2. I have a lump in my breast now.

3. I have had lumps in my breast that I don't have now.

4. This lump:
   went away by itself   was removed by surgery
   [Go to 6]   [Go to 5]
   was removed by some
   other treatment
   [Go to 6]

5. The doctor said this lump
   was malignant (a cancer)
   was benign (not a cancer)
   he didn't say

6. [Women] I have had open sores on my breasts or nipples.

7. [Women] I have had discharges from my nipples.

8. [Women] I have had abcesses in my breasts.

9. This happened right after I had a baby or while I was nursing.

10. I have had an unusual enlargement of one or both breasts.

11. I have had lumps in my armpits.

12. In the past, I have injured my breasts.

13. [Women] I have breastfed one or more of my children.

14. [Women] I know how to examine my own breasts for lumps or tumors.

GYNECOLOGY
(Females only)

1. When I started having my menstrual periods, I was
    9 years old or younger [Go to 3]
    between the ages of 10 and 14 [Go to 3]
    between the ages of 15 and 18 [Go to 3]
    19 years old or older [Go to 3]
    never started having them [Go to 2]

2. I have talked to a doctor about this.
                    [Go to next section]

3. I have gone through the menopause (change of life), or my periods have stopped completely for more than a year.
    No [Go to 4]   Yes [Go to 31]

4. My periods are   regular   irregular

5. I sometimes skip a period.

6. I have a period about every
    2 weeks   6 weeks
    3 weeks   8 weeks
    4 weeks   over 8 weeks
    5 weeks

7. My period usually lasts about
    2 to 3 days   6 to 7 days
    4 to 5 days   over 7 days

8. My last period was about
    I am having my   5 weeks ago
      period now   6 or 7 weeks ago   } [Go to 9]
    1 week ago   } [Go to 9]   8 or 9 weeks ago
    2 weeks ago   10 weeks to a year ago
    3 weeks ago   1 or more years ago [Go to 31]
    4 weeks ago

9. This period was normal for me.

10. I sometimes bleed in between periods.

11. This bleeding is usually
    just before or after my period
    at the halfway point between periods
    during or after sexual relations
    "off and on" anywhere between periods

12. My menstrual flow is   light   average   heavy

13. During a period, the number of sanitary napkins (pads) or tampons I normally use is about

12 or less	3 dozen (36)
2 dozen (24)	4 dozen (48) or more

14. The kind of sanitary napkins (pads) or tampons that I normally use is

regular	double pads
super	pad and tampon at same time

15. I sometimes take a bath towel to bed with me during the second or third day of my period.

16. I have pain (cramps, backache)

with my periods	between my periods
a day or so before my periods	just after my period
	all the time

17. I bleed from my rectum at or around the time of my periods.

18. It is very painful when I move my bowels during my periods.

19. I sometimes have headaches with my periods.

20. I usually get depressed when I have my periods.

21. I swell (feel puffy, bloated) or gain weight with my periods.

22. I think that I am pregnant now.

23. I am upset about this pregnancy.

24. I would like to talk to someone about this.

25. I would like to have more children.

26. I would like some advice about preventing or planning future pregnancies.

27. I do something to prevent pregnancy.

28. I take birth control pills. [Go to 29]
    I use a loop (coil, IUD). [Go to 30]
    I use a diaphragm. [Go to 30]
    I have had my tubes tied. [Go to 30]
    I use some other method of birth control. [Go to 30]

29. All of my pills are the same color.

30. I am now attending a birth control or family planning clinic.
    [Go to 36]

31. My periods stopped

less than a year ago	3 years ago
one year ago	4 years ago
2 years ago	5 or more years ago

32. I have had some bleeding from my vagina since I passed the menopause.

33. I have taken hormones or pills for the menopause (change of life).

34. I am taking these hormones or pills now.

35. I have hot flashes.

36. I have a discharge from my vagina.

37. It is yellow white pink brown

38. It itches.

39. It is watery.

40. It goes on all the time comes and goes

41. My privates (vagina) itch a lot of the time.

42. I have been told I had a pelvic infection.

43. The infection was in my tubes.

44. The infection was right after I was pregnant.

45. I have intercourse or marital relations.

46. I find intercourse or marital relations satisfactory.

47. I reach a climax (orgasm)   never   sometimes   rarely   every time

48. Intercourse or relations are painful for me.

49. I have had a "female" operation of some kind.

50. I have had a D & C.

51. I have had a conization.

52. I have had an operation on my tubes or ovaries.

53. I have had a hysterectomy (have had my uterus removed).

54. The operation was
    through my stomach
    through my vagina

55. I have had vaginal or bladder repair.

56. I have been told that I had fibroids (fireballs, womb stones), or a tumor of the womb.

57. My womb sometimes feels like it is dropping down when I am on my feet.

58. I sometimes can't keep from urinating (passing water) when I cough, sneeze, laugh, or strain.

59. I sometimes feel like I have to urinate and cannot get to the toilet in time.

60. When I am constipated, I have to put my finger in my vagina to move my bowels.

61. I think that I have trouble in my pelvis or some other kind of female trouble.

62. I have been told that I have a positive or a suspicious PAP smear.

63. I have had a PAP smear in the past year.

OBSTETRICAL*
(Females only)

Significance of Response

1. I have been pregnant (count all pregnancies)

Important as to

    Not at all [Go to 2]
    1 time [Go to 5]
    2 times [Go to 5]
    3 times [Go to 5]
    4 times [Go to 5]
    5 times [Go to 5]
    6 times [Go to 5]
    7 times [Go to 5]
    8 times [Go to 5]
    9 or more times
      [Go to 5]

a. high risk of grand multiparity

b. tubal ligation indication

c. together with OB history for habitual aborter

2. I am married.

sociologic insight

    No. [Go to next section]
    Yes. [Go to 3]

3. I haven't had any children because

presence or absence of infertility together with other positive data may point to endometriosis, P.I.D.

    I didn't want any (I use contraceptives or birth control) [Go to next section]
    I tried but couldn't get pregnant [Go to 4]

4. I have been trying to get pregnant for

further modifies question number 3

    1 year or less
    1 to 3 years

* Documentation by Thomas B. Lebherz, M.D., Cleveland Metropolitan General Hospital.

Significance of Response

3 to 5 years
5 to 10 years
10 years or more

[All responses—go to next section]

5. I am pregnant or I think I am pregnant.

will modify date of last menstrual period

No [Go to 19]   Yes [Go to 6]

6. [The patient would now go through this series of questions (6–17) for *each* pregnancy starting with the most recent. When this has been completed, go to 18]

This pregnancy resulted in a

miscarriage [Go to 8]
premature delivery
  [Go to 7]
on-time delivery
  [Go to 9]
overdue delivery
  [Go to 9]

the outcome of previous pregnancies gives information upon which prognosis can be determined with this pregnancy in that

a. repeated miscarriages suggest habitual aborter, incompetent cervix, congenital anomaly of uterus

b. premature deliveries tend to recur if present before. Suspect renal disease, congenital anomaly of uterus, psychiatric problem

c. modifies question number 1

d. post maturity may tend to recur: placental insufficiency

7. The length of this pregnancy was

6 months [Go to 10]
7 months [Go to 10]
8 months [Go to 10]
9 months [Go to 10]

more specifically spells out gross data recorded in question number 6

Significance of Response

8. The length of this pregnancy was

1 month [Go to 17]
2 months [Go to 17]
3 months [Go to 17]
4 months [Go to 17]
5 months [Go to 17]
6 months [Go to 17]
7 months [Go to 17]
8 months [Go to 17]

more specifically spells out gross data recorded in question number 6

9. The length of this pregnancy was

8 months [Go to 10]
9 months [Go to 10]
10 months [Go to 10]
11 months [Go to 10]

more specifically spells out gross data recorded in question number 6

10. The length of labor before this delivery was

less than one hour
1 to 8 hours
9 to 18 hours
19 hours or longer

the length of labor with previous deliveries is applicable to prognosis with regard to delivery of present pregnancy

11. The type of delivery was

normal (without forceps)
   [Go to 13]
with forceps [Go to 13]
through my stomach (Cesarian section) [Go to 12]
I don't remember
   [Go to 13]

further aids in prognosticating outcome of present pregnancy

Significance of Response

12. I had a Cesarian delivery because

I was bleeding too much
[Go to 14]
my afterbirth separated
[Go to 14]
I was too small [Go to 14]
the baby was in the wrong
position [Go to 14]
the baby was in trouble
[Go to 14]
I had kidney trouble
[Go to 14]
my labor was too long
[Go to 14]
my womb wouldn't dilate
[Go to 14]
I don't know or can't
remember [Go to 14]
I have diabetes [Go to 14]

the historical indication for a
previous C-section gives insight
into type and degree of complication of a previous section and may
play a part in deciding to deliver
this pregnancy vaginally

13. The way the baby came
out was

head first
rear-end or feet first
don't remember

breech deliveries tend to recur;
breech deliveries followed by late
abortions may suggest cervical in-
competence. Also one would tend
to identify a difficult breech as a
cause for a previous prenatal death

14. The type of anesthesia I had
for this delivery was

local
spinal
gas
none (natural
childbirth)
other
don't remember

this helps in deciding what anesthesia to use with the present
pregnancy

Significance of Response

15. This baby was born alive.

outcome of previous pregnancy, especially as far as stillbirths are concerned, is especially important when interested in diabetes, post maturity or essential hypertension

16. This baby's weight was

less than 5½ pounds
5½ to 9 pounds
greater than 9 pounds
I don't remember

weight of previous babies has a definite bearing on the present pregnancy, for instance in a known small pelvis, possibility of gestational diabetes, etc.

17. The complications I had with this pregnancy were

none [Go to 6 for next previous pregnancy]
anemia
jaundice
kidney infection
thrombophlebitis
toxemia (high blood pressure)
done [Go to 6 for next previous pregnancy]

complications of previous pregnancies, tend to recur, especially those listed, and would indicate treatment or close observation

18. I have had twins or triplets. [Go to 25]

multiple pregnancy tends to recur or may be related to clinical treatment

19. When I was pregnant I had high blood pressure.

toxemia with a previous pregnancy tends to recur in future pregnancies, as does essential hypertension

20. The number of living children I have now is

no children   5 children
1 child   6 children
2 children   7 children
3 children   8 children
4 children   9 or more children

confirms data relating to perinatal mortality and may play a part in a tubal ligation decision

Significance of Response

21. The number of children that
    I have had that have been
    born alive is

no children	5 children	when cross checked with
1 child	6 children	questions 1–9 & 20, pro-
2 children	7 children	vides an overall picture
3 children	8 or more	of this patient's obstetri-
4 children	children	cal past history which is

very important to this
pregnancy from the
standpoint of abortion,
prematurity, prognosis
in the face of H.B.P.,
diabetes, post maturity
or congenital anomalies
of the uterus

22. The number of stillborn
    babies that I have had is

none	5 stillborn babies	
1 stillborn baby	6 stillborn babies	
2 stillborn babies	7 or more still-	same as question
3 stillborn babies	born babies	number 21
4 stillborn babies		

23. The number of miscarriages
    that I have had is

none	5 miscarriages	
1 miscarriage	6 miscarriages	
2 miscarriages	7 miscarriages	same as question
3 miscarriages	8 or more mis-	number 21
4 miscarriages	carriages	

Significance of Response

24. The number of premature
    babies that I have had is

none	5 premature babies	
1 premature baby		
2 premature babies	6 premature babies	same as question number 21
3 premature babies	7 premature babies	
4 premature babies	8 or more premature babies	

25. The number of children that
    I have adopted is

no children	5 children	
1 child	6 children	
2 children	7 children	same as question number 21
3 children	8 or more children	
4 children		

26. I have had a baby that weighed over 9 pounds.

35% of women who deliver children in excess of 9 lbs. will develop clinical diabetes or will develop gestational diabetes with subsequent pregnancy

27. I have had a baby that weighed less than 5½ pounds.

premature babies tend to recur; at the same time this query alerts the physician to be wary of uterine anomalies, incompetent cervix

28. I have had a blood transfusion during a delivery.

anemia with previous pregnancy or an acute blood-loss problem, either of which may tend to recur

29. I breast fed one or more of my children.

insight as to outcome if patient desires to breast feed. Some relationship to breast cancer—*but variably significant*

Significance of Response

30. When I was pregnant I had convulsions.

convulsions suggesting eclampsia or epilepsy during previous delivery warn that both entities may recur

31. When I was pregnant I had albumin in my urine.

albumin in the urine suggests renal disease or toxemia

32. When I was pregnant I had sugar in my urine.

sugar in the urine in past suggests indication for I.V. G.T.T.

33. When I was pregnant I was anemic.

anemia past history indicates need for close study of the problem with this pregnancy to include repeat studies sooner

34. When I was pregnant I had jaundice.

idiopathic or drug-related liver problems, especially common during pregnancy and tending to recur, must be considered

35. When I was pregnant I had generalized itching.

same as question number 34

36. I had other illnesses during pregnancy.

many diseases may recur with this pregnancy, or sequelae of previous diseases may complicate this pregnancy, such as, thrombophlebitis, urinary tract infections, asthma, etc.

37. I have had a baby who had to have a transfusion after birth.

relates to anticipated outcome of this pregnancy with relation to Rh disease, necessitating closer observation prenatally and close attention postnatally to the baby

38. This was an Rh factor baby.

same as question number 37

39. I have had a baby who had to stay in the hospital for longer than 2 weeks after he was born.

same as question number 37

Significance of Response

40. This was due to yellow jaundice.

same as question number 37

41. I have had a baby who had to have an operation during the first 2 years of his life.

congenital anomalies needing operative correction can be suspected

42. I have had a baby who died before he was 1 year old.

congenital enzymatic disease with CNA involvement tends to recur in the same family

43. Right after I was pregnant I had an infection in my urine.

prior urinary tract infections tend to recur ante partum with subsequent pregnancy

44. Right after I was pregnant I had an infection in my breasts.

45. Right after I was pregnant I had excessive bleeding or hemorrhage.

postpartum hemorrhage tends to recur

46. Right after I was pregnant I had thrombophlebitis (infection in my veins).

postpartum thrombophlebitis in the past tends to recur in future pregnancies

47. Right after I was pregnant I had a nervous breakdown.

postpartum psychosis tends to recur

GENITOURINARY

1. In the past year I have had problems or trouble with my bladder or with urinating (passing water).

2. When I pass water there is pain or burning.

3. I sometimes lose control of my bladder.

4. I have trouble starting my stream.

5. My bladder doesn't seem to empty most of the time.

6. My urine dribbles.

7. My urine has been bloody or coffee-colored.

8. My urine turns red, black or dark colored when left standing.

9. I have been told that I had protein or albumin in my urine.

10. I often get up in the middle of the night to urinate.

11. I usually have to get up

    once a night   three times a night
    twice a night   more than three times a night

12. In the past, I have had sand in my urine.

13. A doctor told me that I had kidney or bladder stones.

14. The stones left by way of my stream (came out when I passed water).

15. I had surgery for these stones.

16. A doctor has told me that I had a kidney disease.

17. A doctor has told me that I had a kidney or bladder infection.

18. I have had these infections often.

19. [Women] I had this infection during or after pregnancy.

20. I have had syphilis or bad blood.

21. I have had gonorrhea or the clap.

22. I have had a bladder or kidney operation.

23. I had kidney trouble as a child.

24. I have had X rays taken of my kidneys.

25. I think I have some sort of kidney trouble.

26. I have sex problems:

    and would like to discuss them
    but do not wish to discuss them with anybody
    no, I don't have any sex problems

(Remaining questions for men only)

27. The size or force of my urine stream has gotten smaller.

28. I have had trouble with my prostate gland.

29. A doctor told me that I had an enlarged prostate.

30. A doctor told me that I had cancer of the prostate.

31. A doctor told me that I had an infected prostate.

32. I had surgery for prostate trouble.

33. I have taken hormone medicine for prostate trouble.

34. I have been having troubles with my penis (privates, male organ).

35. I have had hard lumps or sores on my penis.

36. I have had an abnormal discharge from my penis.

37. I have had a loss of sex interest.

38. I have had a loss of sex ability or nature.

39. I have or have had a rupture or hernia.

40. I have been having trouble with my scrotum (sac) or my testicles (seeds).

41. I have a painful infection there.

42. My testicles have become larger.

43. My testicles have become stone hard.

44. My scrotum (sac) is swollen.

45. I have been circumcised.

46. I have had my sperm tubes tied (sterilization).

NEUROLOGY*

Significance of Response

1. I have bad headaches.

2. These headaches are a real   no specificity
   problem.

3. They are getting worse or   worsening disease
   more frequent.

---

* Documentation of neurology questions by Fred Hochberg, M.D., Cleveland Metropolitan General Hospital.

Significance of Response

4. I get these headaches about

   every day [Go to 5] tension, cluster†

   three or four times a week tension
   [Go to 5]

   once a week [Go to 5] migraine‡

   once a month or less non-specific
   [Go to 5]

   they are continuous (I tension
   always have a headache)
   [Go to 7]

5. These headaches usually last

   less than 1 hour ⎫ retrobulbar cephalgia
   several hours   ⎬ greater than 6 hours: ↑
   several days   ⎭ likelihood neurological
                      disease; structural;
                      abnormal sinus; teeth,
                      or vascular

6. These headaches usually occur

   in the morning tumor, ↑ intracranial pressure

   during the daytime tension

   in the evening tension

   different times during r/o cluster
   the day

7. These headaches awake me ? tumor, subarachnoid
   at night. bleeding

8. These headaches make my ? vascular, non-specific
   head throb

9. I have had this trouble with
   headaches for

   a week or less ⎫
   several weeks ⎬
   several months ⎬ symptom duration
   a year or more ⎬
   5 years or more ⎭

---

† Cluster: regular unilateral headache near temple or eye, often associated with lacrimation, occurring in definite clusters; periods of varying frequency and usually shorter than 2 hours in length.

‡ Migraine: familial paroxysmal unilateral headache preceded by scotomata,

Significance of Response

10. I feel nauseated (sick to my stomach) or I vomit when I have these headaches.

symptom severity; suggest neuro basis, especially vascular

11. Tension or nervousness triggers my headaches.

tension, migraine

12. I have a feeling of a tight band around my head.

? hysterical

13. The position my body is in affects my headaches.

? paraventricular tumor, migraine, intracranial headache

14. I sometimes have a change in eyesight when I have these headaches.

vertebral insufficiency, migraine scotoma. photophobia: migraine. dimness: ↑ CSF pressure.

15. These headaches usually occur in the same place every time

localization

16. They usually occur

in the back of my head or neck

tension or ↑ BP, basilar artery vascular disease, posterior fossa

in my forehead

posterior fossa, ↑ pressure unilateral = cluster

near my temples

tension, ↑ BP, arteritis, otitis, toothache

above one or both eyes

increased intracranial pressure, glaucoma, subarachnoid hemorrhage, sinusitis, cluster

on top of my head

subarachnoid hemorrhage

all over

non-specific (increased CSF pressure, tension, post LP headache)

---

associated with nausea and vomiting and neurologic changes contralateral to headache and worsened by stress. Lasts less than 12 hours.

Significance of Response

17. They usually occur

    on my left side
    on my right side   localization, cluster (unilateral),
    on both sides   migraine, tooth, sinus, otitis
    in the middle

18. These headaches keep me   cluster, subarachnoid bleeding
    awake at night.

19. I can usually tell when I am   tension, migraine
    going to get a headache.

20. Other people in my family   tension, migraine
    have severe headaches.

21. I often have dizzy spells.

22. I have a feeling of light-   ? value
    headedness with these
    spells.

23. I have a feeling of a whirling   vertigo
    sensation with these spells.

24. Objects sometimes seem to   ? value
    rotate or move when I
    have these spells.

25. These spells often come with   Ménière's, drug systemic
    ringing or noises in my   lupus erythematous
    ears, or in the room.

26. I often feel nauseated (sick   basilar insufficiency,
    to my stomach) or vomit   Ménière's disease
    with these spells.

Significance of Response

27. I have had these dizzy
    spells for

    a week or less   basilar insufficiency,
                              short history

    several weeks   )
    several months   }   Ménière's, long history
    a year or more   }   (may be < ½ hr)
    5 years or more   )

28. I find it very hard to walk   Ménière's, basilar insufficiency.
    when I'm having one of   true vertigo: ataxic. psycho-
    these spells.   neurotic: dizzy

29. I am dizzy all the time.   ? psychiatric

    No [Go to 30]
    Yes [Go to 31]

30.   These attacks of dizziness
      usually last

      less than 1 hour
      less than 6 hours   vascular disease
      less than 12 hours
      less than one day   Ménière's
      more than one day   Ménière's

31. I have to remain still during   severity (vertigo)
    an attack.

32. These dizzy spells are made   Ménière's, greater basilar
    worse by moving my head.   insufficiency, inseverity

33. I have noticed a peculiar,   uncinate seizures
    strange taste or smell for
    a few minutes which I
    could not understand.

34. I have had convulsions or fits   non-specific questioning for
    (include psychomotor   seizures. may not
    seizures) after age 5.   exclude ↓ BP, ↓ glucose

Significance of Response

35. I have had blackout spells.

36. I have had seizures.

37. I have had falling out spells.

38. I have had epilepsy.   diagnosis specific
    [If "no" to all above 5
    questions, go to 50]

39. I can tell when I am going to   aura or predisposing
    have one of these   symptoms ↓ BP, ↓ glucose
    occurrences.

40. These happenings are usually
    preceded by

    dizziness
    nausea
    headaches
    paleness
    none of these

41. During attacks, I breathe   hyperventilation syndrome
    quickly and notice
    tingling around my mouth.

42. These attacks sometimes   non-specific ↓ glucose,
    occur during the night.   r/o ↓ BP, seizures

43. These attacks sometimes   seizures
    occur when I am lying flat.

44. I shake when I have these   motor seizure
    spells.

45. I shake
       on my left side   ⎫
       on my right side ⎬   localizing motor strip
       all over   ⎭

Significance of Response

46. I sometimes bite my tongue or injure myself when I have one of these spells.   epilepsy specific

47. I sometimes lose my water when I have one of these spells.   epilepsy

48. These spells are usually followed by a time of confusion, headaches, or drowsiness.   non-specific

49. I have had these spells for

    a week or less
    several weeks
    several months }   time specificity
    a year or more
    5 years or more

50. I have had a stroke.

51. I have trouble moving my arms or legs.   ? Todd paralysis (post convulsion paralysis)

52. The trouble is in my

    arms
    legs }   seizure localization; stroke or paresis
    arms and legs

53. The trouble is on

    my right side
    my left side }   localization
    both sides

54. I often have uncontrolled movement of my arms and legs.   seizure or automatic movement

55. I am awkward so I can't do things like button buttons or walk very well.   decreased motor/sensory function, non-specific

Significance of Response

56. The trouble is in my
    arms and hands
    arms, hands, legs, and feet } localization
    legs and feet

57. The trouble is mainly on
    my right side
    my left side
    both sides

58. I have numbness or tingling   paresthesias, non-specific
    of my hands or feet.

59. I have had this numbness
    or tingling for
    a week or less
    several weeks
    several months }   time duration
    a year or more
    5 years or more

60. I have had difficulty speaking   dysarthria/aphasia
    or pronouncing words.

61. I have sometimes lost the   anarthria/aphasia
    ability to speak for a few
    minutes.

62. People have noticed a   dysarthria/aphasia
    change in the way I speak.

63. I have sometimes missed a   expressive aphasia
    common, everyday word
    when I knew what I
    wanted to say.

64. I sometimes have a hard time   receptive difficulty
    understanding words.

65. I sometimes have a hard time   ? expressive difficulty,
    making people understand   non-specific
    what I mean.

	Significance of Response
66. I often forget things.	memory, aphasia
67. I forget things that have happened in the past.	long-term memory
68. I forget things that have happened recently.	short-term memory
69. I am much more sensitive to pain all over one side of my body than on the other side.	hypesthesia

PSYCHIATRY

*1. There are times when I cry a lot and can't control myself.

2. There are times when I feel very lonely so that I cannot go on living.

3. I stay alone a lot and avoid people.

4. I see things or animals or people around me that others do not see.

*5. Some of the time I wish I were dead.

6. I find it impossible to really enjoy anything.

*7. I have thought about committing suicide (taking my own life).

*8. In the past, I have attempted suicide (tried to take my own life).

9. I have the wanderlust and am never happy unless I am roaming or traveling about.

10. I often feel terribly nervous or afraid without knowing why.

11. I often get so frightened that I am afraid to go out of my home alone.

12. I believe I am a condemned person.

---

* Indicates screening questions for administration of a Minnesota Multiphasic Personality Inventory (MMPI). Alcohol questions in patient profile are also considered part of this section.

*13. I sometimes have strange or crazy thoughts that I cannot get rid of.

*14. I often feel that people are talking about me, working against me, or are out to get me.

15. I commonly hear voices without knowing where they come from.

16. I often have trouble controlling my temper.

17. I am afraid of using sharp instruments or tools (like a knife).

18. Someone has control over my mind.

19. I have a lot of accidents at home or at work.

20. I feel anxious about something or someone almost all the time.

21. There are people at home or at work that keep me constantly upset.

22. I have trouble sleeping.

23. I have trouble falling asleep.

24. I often wake up in the middle of the night and can't get back to sleep.

25. I always wake up very early in the morning, even if I am very tired.

*26. In the past I have felt extremely depressed or hopeless.

27. Peculiar odors come to me at times.

28. I take tranquilizers or nerve pills regularly.

29. I use narcotics (dope) or some other drug to get high on.

30. I have been hooked on drugs.

31. It seems like everything has always gone wrong for me.

*32. I find it difficult to talk or think about my sexual feelings.

33. I have problems in my sex life.

*34. I worry about these problems a great deal.

35. I am less interested in sex or enjoy it less now than I used to.

36. [Women] I have had mental troubles due to the change or menopause.

37. I have often feared that there was something wrong with my mind.

38. A family history of mental illness is one of my worries.

*39. I have had a nervous breakdown.

*40. I have been hospitalized because of a nervous breakdown or any nerve problem.

41. I feel that a psychiatrist could help me.

42. I feel that sometimes I have too many responsibilities.

43. I often daydream about being another person.

44. I think that I am usually very tense.

45. My living conditions are below the standards I have been accustomed to.

46. My living conditions are so bad, it keeps me upset.

APPENDIX B

Recording Physical
*Examinations by Computer**

Private practitioners, subspecialty clinics, whole institutions, and even medical supply houses have created a wide variety of materials in an attempt to formalize the recording of physical examinations. As with all recording systems, the format has varied widely according to the purpose at hand. Thus we find a multitude of forms available on which the physician is encouraged to make specific disease or organ-system-oriented observations in a subspecialty area or simply to record his general examination within a standardized framework. The very diversity of these materials reflects a nearly limitless variety in clinical situations and methodologies.

Any attempt to create a unified system must take the diversity of medical settings into account and prove itself adaptable to each. A system that functions well only in a limited number of situations will clearly be of very little value.

Most complaints regarding the deficiencies of physical examination forms involve the *completeness* with which data may be recorded, the *narrowness of scope* of the form, the difficulty in *adapting the same form*

---

* The displays used in this appendix were developed by Robert Putsch, M.D., and the commentary is by Dr. Putsch. The completed displays for the entire physical examination were the result of the combined efforts of many on the staff of the Cleveland Metropolitan General Hospital and will be published as a separate manual.

229

to a wide variety of clinical settings, and, finally, the *lack of flexibility* in the form that would permit an expansion in the format of the examination and an accommodation of the resulting additional commentary.

It is clear that the form per se does little to guarantee thoroughness in recording a physical examination. It is as easy to skip areas in which observations are requested on a form as it is to omit them when one begins with a blank page and neglects a major category (chest, heart, abdomen, rectal, and genitalia.) A branching TV terminal, such as has earlier been described, can be employed for recording physical examination data. It employs a multiple branching system that initially confronts the physician with those information items that are felt to be essential in a proper physical examination of all patients and branches to allow either highly specific commentary, when the choice among items needs further clarification, or to by-pass items that become irrelevant on the basis of a previously recorded observation (e.g., to by-pass behavior characteristics in a comatose patient). Not only are the physician's comments structured, but he must complete comments on each portion of the examination before he is allowed to progress to the next. A rectal examination, for instance, even if "not performed," must be recorded as such prior to progressing to the neurological exam that follows.

As designed for use in the TV-terminal type of recording system, the physical examination reproduced below has a framework similar to that outlined in many physical diagnosis books. A successful examination system must be highly flexible and complete. The key to easy accessibility in clinical settings lies in the nature of the major categories and subdivisions under which observations are recorded. Figure B-1 represents the "General Description" section of the physical examination as it is set up on the TV terminal system at Cleveland Metropolitan General Hospital. Two points are worth noting:

1. The material recorded in the statement can be varied to meet particular needs, whether of a geriatrics unit, an emergency room, or a well-baby clinic. However, once the basic statement is established, a choice at each step must be made by the physician each time he uses the system. If he does not make a choice, he cannot continue, and a degree of thoroughness in establishing the record is thereby guaranteed that cannot be achieved by the use of a form.

2. Most physicians would include in the record of their examination a short comment regarding the mental status of the patient. We feel,

however, that mental status constitutes a category of enough importance to warrant its definition as a major subdivision of the branching display. When the category of mental status is defined in this way, the physician first makes choices from standard displays and thus records a general mental-status statement. If he feels a more complete commentary is necessary, he simply enters a more intricately branching series of specific inquiries in the basic format and so generates a more thorough statement in this area.

Figure B-2, which represents the first displays of the external eye examination, provides a sharp contrast to the display in Fig. B-1. The former display illustrates the depth and completeness of a branching system and its potential for overcoming the narrow scope of printed forms. The numerous satellite displays of Fig. B-2, connected by "loops" of varying lengths, are the "hidden" selections that allow a wide variety of refined statements to be recorded about the external eye alone. Contrast this refinement to the more conventional approach of the mark-sense printed form.* The "eye" portion of an examination prepared in this fashion is reproduced in Fig. B-3.† An obvious problem is apparent: Choices are limited and incomplete. Furthermore, all possible choices must be represented at once, and the necessity to present all possible variants can be terribly cumbersome and confusing. Corrections or additions to the mark-sense examination require not only that the individual page be changed but that the material which follows be displaced, requiring reprogramming for the scanning device.

The step-by-step progression through the entire examination occurs only when a complete examination is to be recorded, as in a new inpatient or outpatient evaluation. The framework of the entire examination can be utilized as an index in those instances in which portions of

---

* A mark-sense sheet is similar to a testing form in which answers are entered by marks penciled into the appropriate spaces. It is "read" by an optical scanning device which records positive responses on a punch card.

† This examination was designed in 1967 by Charles Burger, M.D., at Cleveland Metropolitan General Hospital. It compares favorably in its completeness with similar examinations prepared at a number of other centers. Dr. Burger's initial efforts in computerizing the physical examination (done in conjunction with Mr. Eugene Lovesay and utilizing an IBM 1440 with optical scan sheets) formed the basis of our present program. The experience gained in using his forms in a clinical setting has been invaluable in our current developmental efforts.

FIGURE B-1. This figure represents the "General Appearance" section of the physical examination. Each "box" is a single TV terminal display. The series begins at #1 in the upper left corner and ends with #12. In order to write a description of this patient, the physician simply touches the TV-tube terminal at the point of appropriate selection. The machine responds by changing from one display to the next so rapidly that one is barely aware of the change of frames on the screen. Note that the sequence which the machine will follow depends entirely upon the choice of statements. Thus a choice of "unresponsive" at #7 leads directly to #12. The "General Appearance" section follows the vital signs, and once it is completed the physician touches either "none of the above" or "continue," both of which are on display #12. He will immediately continue with the skin examination at this point. The title for the first display is recorded automatically, along with the modifying statement selected by the physician. Thus a touch of the finger would write, "the patient is a chronically ill." The material is printed in final form as a complete sentence. Example: "The patient is an acutely ill, obese, Caucasian male, aged 54 years. Responsive, not fully cooperative, being too ill, and can care for self. Currently requires GI aids, colostomy." A 29-word statement is thus generated by touching the terminal only 13 times, faster than the material can be written with a pen.

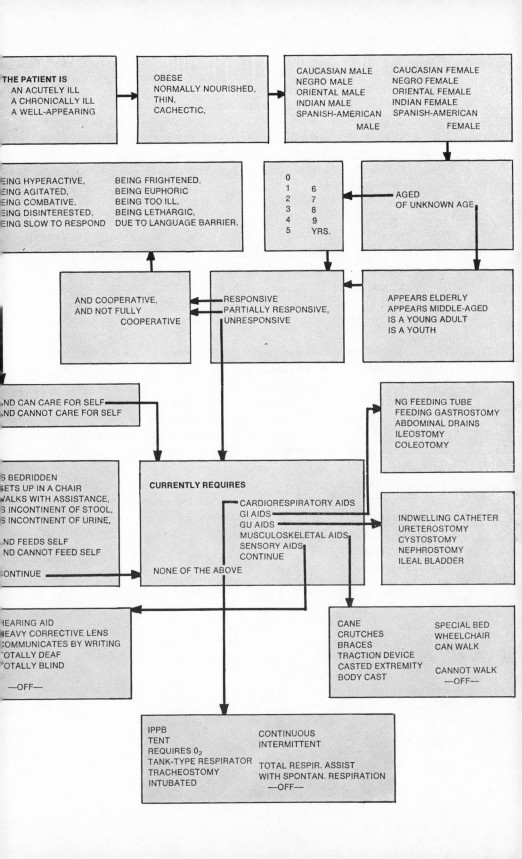

THE PATIENT IS
   AN ACUTELY ILL
   A CHRONICALLY ILL
   A WELL-APPEARING

OBESE
NORMALLY NOURISHED,
THIN,
CACHECTIC,

CAUCASIAN MALE   CAUCASIAN FEMALE
NEGRO MALE   NEGRO FEMALE
ORIENTAL MALE   ORIENTAL FEMALE
INDIAN MALE   INDIAN FEMALE
SPANISH-AMERICAN   SPANISH-AMERICAN
            MALE   FEMALE

EING HYPERACTIVE,   BEING FRIGHTENED,
EING AGITATED,   BEING EUPHORIC
EING COMBATIVE,   BEING TOO ILL,
EING DISINTERESTED,   BEING LETHARGIC,
EING SLOW TO RESPOND   DUE TO LANGUAGE BARRIER,

0
1   6
2   7
3   8
4   9
5   YRS.

AGED
OF UNKNOWN AGE,

AND COOPERATIVE,
AND NOT FULLY
      COOPERATIVE

RESPONSIVE
PARTIALLY RESPONSIVE,
UNRESPONSIVE

APPEARS ELDERLY
APPEARS MIDDLE-AGED
IS A YOUNG ADULT
IS A YOUTH

ND CAN CARE FOR SELF
ND CANNOT CARE FOR SELF

NG FEEDING TUBE
FEEDING GASTROSTOMY
ABDOMINAL DRAINS
ILEOSTOMY
COLEOTOMY

S BEDRIDDEN
ETS UP IN A CHAIR
WALKS WITH ASSISTANCE,
S INCONTINENT OF STOOL,
S INCONTINENT OF URINE,

ND FEEDS SELF
ND CANNOT FEED SELF

ONTINUE

CURRENTLY REQUIRES

CARDIORESPIRATORY AIDS
GI AIDS
GU AIDS
MUSCULOSKELETAL AIDS
SENSORY AIDS
CONTINUE

NONE OF THE ABOVE

INDWELLING CATHETER
URETEROSTOMY
CYSTOSTOMY
NEPHROSTOMY
ILEAL BLADDER

HEARING AID
EAVY CORRECTIVE LENS
COMMUNICATES BY WRITING
OTALLY DEAF
OTALLY BLIND

—OFF—

CANE   SPECIAL BED
CRUTCHES   WHEELCHAIR
BRACES   CAN WALK
TRACTION DEVICE
CASTED EXTREMITY   CANNOT WALK
BODY CAST   —OFF—

IPPB
TENT   CONTINUOUS
REQUIRES 0₂   INTERMITTENT
TANK-TYPE RESPIRATOR
TRACHEOSTOMY   TOTAL RESPIR. ASSIST
INTUBATED   WITH SPONTAN. RESPIRATION
                         —OFF—

single sections, as opposed to an entire examination, are to be recorded. One might, for instance, want to include parts of the vital signs, neck, chest, heart, and lower extremity examinations in a progress note about a congestive failure problem. The physician would simply "enter" the examination through the index at these five categories, make his comments, and quickly come back out of the physical examination portion altogether. Through the use of an index of this sort, the physical examination portion of clinic and emergency room notes, progress notes, and the like can be rapidly recorded. In those areas of extremely common problems, such as minor trauma or warts in the dermatology clinics, short "loops" can be arranged for rapid access and the preparation of brief but concise notes. Subspecialists and teaching services may find it useful to establish their own loops, or paths, through the framework to insure a base line of material that will always be covered by their consultants.

The employment of the examination framework as an index allows a degree of flexibility of another important kind. As experience with the examination builds, individual areas can easily be rearranged and simple loops or even major subdivisions can be added or removed at no penalty to the structure as a whole. The perfection of the system depends, of course, on a willingness to update and improve it. Displays can be altered in a matter of minutes. The display sequences may be thought of as a deck of cards in which single cards may be readily inserted, from which they may be removed, or within which they may be altered without disturbing the overall structure. Repeated series of examinations will permit the correlation of large numbers of clinical encounters and thus permit accurate generalizations in a field that has been full of vagaries and assumptions.

FIGURE B-2. The first display in a series of four subdivisions that comprise the eye examination. It consists of a single central display and a large number of branching "loops." The user is never aware of the numerous branched pathways until he chooses to make a comment that will lead him into one of them. Unlike the procedure for example in Fig. B-1, the procedure here does not force the user to enter any of the minor circuits; he does so only by choice. For example, the eye signs in an alcoholic patient might be described as follows: "EYE, external exam, abn. movement (or deviation), nystagmus, horizontal, fine, on lat. gaze, both eyes." Note that three choices were selected on the last display of the series. The displays with an "—OFF—" permit multiple choices, the physician making as many touches as necessary prior to moving on to the next area. When he is through with the display, however, he goes on to the next major subdivision. After touching "both eyes," he touches "—OFF—" again and proceeds to the next part of the eye exam.

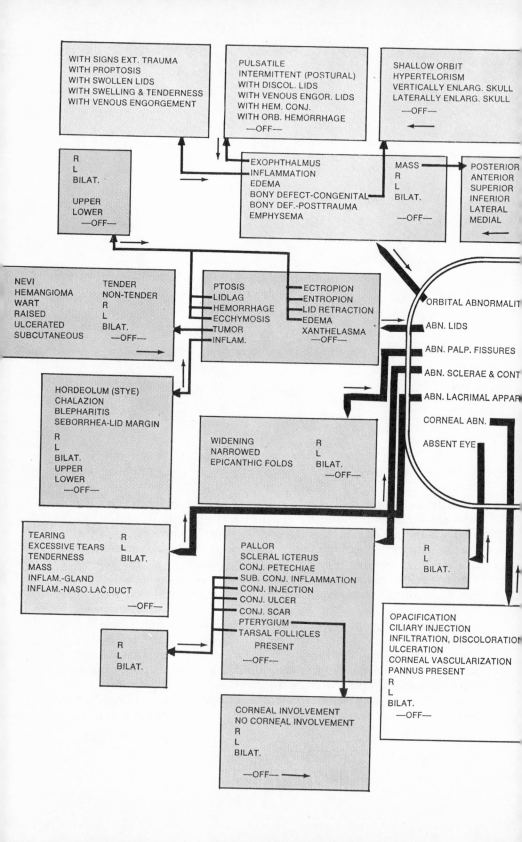

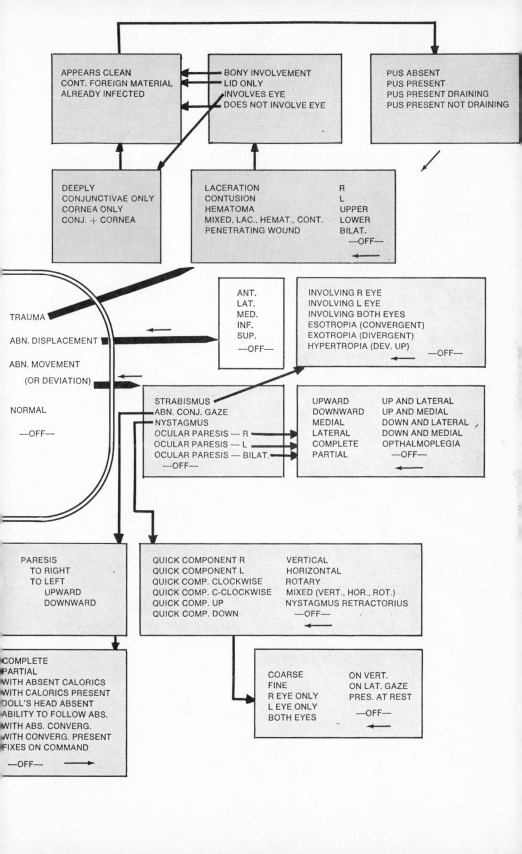

APPEARS CLEAN
CONT. FOREIGN MATERIAL
ALREADY INFECTED

BONY INVOLVEMENT
LID ONLY
INVOLVES EYE
DOES NOT INVOLVE EYE

PUS ABSENT
PUS PRESENT
PUS PRESENT DRAINING
PUS PRESENT NOT DRAINING

DEEPLY
CONJUNCTIVAE ONLY
CORNEA ONLY
CONJ. + CORNEA

LACERATION   R
CONTUSION   L
HEMATOMA   UPPER
MIXED, LAC., HEMAT., CONT.   LOWER
PENETRATING WOUND   BILAT.
                          —OFF—

TRAUMA

ABN. DISPLACEMENT

ABN. MOVEMENT
  (OR DEVIATION)

NORMAL

  —OFF—

ANT.
LAT.
MED.
INF.
SUP.
—OFF—

INVOLVING R EYE
INVOLVING L EYE
INVOLVING BOTH EYES
ESOTROPIA (CONVERGENT)
EXOTROPIA (DIVERGENT)
HYPERTROPIA (DEV. UP)
                    —OFF—

STRABISMUS
ABN. CONJ. GAZE
NYSTAGMUS
OCULAR PARESIS — R
OCULAR PARESIS — L
OCULAR PARESIS — BILAT.
  —OFF—

UPWARD   UP AND LATERAL
DOWNWARD   UP AND MEDIAL
MEDIAL   DOWN AND LATERAL
LATERAL   DOWN AND MEDIAL
COMPLETE   OPTHALMOPLEGIA
PARTIAL   —OFF—

PARESIS
   TO RIGHT
   TO LEFT
      UPWARD
      DOWNWARD

QUICK COMPONENT R   VERTICAL
QUICK COMPONENT L   HORIZONTAL
QUICK COMP. CLOCKWISE   ROTARY
QUICK COMP. C-CLOCKWISE MIXED (VERT., HOR., ROT.)
QUICK COMP. UP   NYSTAGMUS RETRACTORIUS
QUICK COMP. DOWN   —OFF—

COMPLETE
PARTIAL
WITH ABSENT CALORICS
WITH CALORICS PRESENT
DOLL'S HEAD ABSENT
ABILITY TO FOLLOW ABS.
WITH ABS. CONVERG.
WITH CONVERG. PRESENT
FIXES ON COMMAND

  —OFF—

COARSE   ON VERT.
FINE   ON LAT. GAZE
R EYE ONLY   PRES. AT REST
L EYE ONLY   —OFF—
BOTH EYES

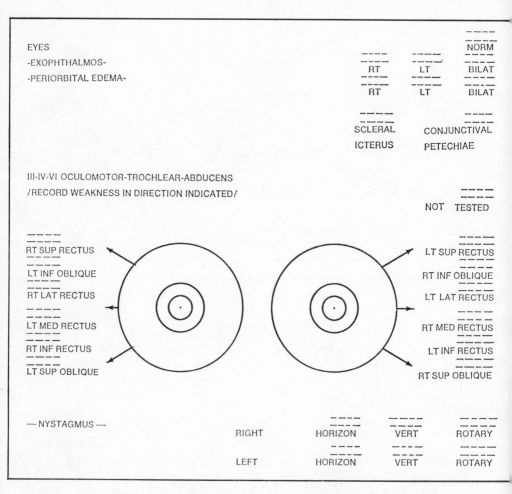

FIGURE B-3. This is the external eye portion of an eye examination prepared on a mark-sense format. Positive responses are recorded as horizontal pencil marks in the appropriate blanks.

APPENDIX C

Example of a
Problem-Oriented Summary
Prepared for Grand Rounds

This was the 2nd CMGH [Cleveland Metropolitan General Hospital] admission for this 4-month-old white male with hepatomegaly.

PROBLEM #1. PERSISTENT NASAL CONGESTION

SUBJECTIVE: The mother describes "trouble breathing" since the newborn period. Pregnancy was uneventful except for 2 or 3 isolated episodes of spotting in the 2nd trimester; she had a seizure sometime during the 24 hours before delivery but details are not known.

At three months of age, the patient was admitted to a West Virginia hospital for "double pneumonia." He was brought here after an indeterminate stay in that hospital and found to have no pneumonia but persistent nasal congestion. The congestion of the nose persisted during this hospitalization, was unresponsive to nasal constrictors, and did not interfere with feeding.

OBJECTIVE: Three weeks prior to admission the patient took his feedings well but with much choking and coughing. Chest X ray then showed a minimal enlargement of the right hilum. He remained afebrile. Culture of the nose during this admission showed heavy Hemophilus influenzae and light alpha Strep. Chest X ray will be described below under diagnosis #5.

THERAPEUTIC: Neo-synephrine nose drops were to no avail. Antibiotics as under #5.

PROBLEM #2. FEEDING PROBLEM

SUBJECTIVE: He regurgitated after feedings since about one month of age; this continued until this admission, though was somewhat decreased by soybean milk. The parents were told after birth to feed the baby hourly for 2–3 weeks as he was "dehydrated." The regurgitation has always occurred within 30 minutes of feeding and is always undigested food. There is no suggestion of colic; he has 2–3 formed, brown, not foul-smelling stools per day.

Regurgitation was observed on only two occasions during this hospitalization; otherwise appetite was excellent and feeding vigorous.

OBJECTIVE: Birth weight was 2750 grams. Three weeks prior to admission he was at the 25th percentile for weight; on admission was less than a 10th percentile; on discharge was exactly at the 10th percentile. Length is at the 10th percentile, and head circumference at the 25th. Sweat chloride one week prior to admission was 17 mEq/L.

THERAPEUTIC: Baker's milk for the first three weeks of life; then a formula made of 21 oz of evaporated milk, 7 oz water, plus Karo syrup. Switched to soybean milk in the Outpatient Department two weeks prior to admission.

PROBLEM #3. GLYCOGEN STORAGE DISEASE, TYPE UNKNOWN

SUBJECTIVE: No episodes suggestive of hypoglycemia have been observed; a gradually increasing abdominal girth was noticed for the two weeks prior to admission.

OBJECTIVE: Several examinations in the Outpatient Clinic by several examiners during the month prior to admission did not reveal hepatomegaly. However, the day of admission, the liver was found to be 7–8 cm below the right costal margin, extending across the midline.

Studies on admission included: Examination of the stool showed no reducing substances, a pH of 6, and an increase in muscle fiber but no increased fat. Glucagon tolerance test was performed after a 10-hour fast and the curve was essentially flat; the fasting sugar was 52, and the blood glucose reached a high of 66 at one hour after the injection of glucagon. Two days prior to discharge, a galactose test followed by a glucagon tolerance test was performed. Percutaneous liver biopsy was performed before the above test with the following interpretation: H and E stained sections showed large unstained cytoplasmic vacuoles in the liver cells. Many liver cells did not contain vacuoles but the cytoplasm appeared granular. Sections stained with PAS [paramino salicylic acid] showed PAS-positive granules in the cytoplasm without staining of the large vacuoles. PAS staining of the granules was blocked by diastase digestion, and alcohol-fixed sections showed better preservation of the granules which were thought to represent glycogen. Small PAS-positive intranuclear granules, liable to diastase digestion, were identified in a few cells. There was no fibrosis seen. Diagnosis was "glycogenosis and fat accumulation of liver, consistent with glycogen storage disease." Sections of liver show striking vacuolization of hepatic cell cytoplasms, presumably due to fat deposition. Liver cytoplasm contains abundant PAS-positive granules which are removed with prior diastase digestion. The histology is most suggestive of type 1 glycogen storage disease. Type 4 glycogen storage disease is ruled out microscopically. Type 3 glycogen storage disease (debrancher deficiency) and the three different phosphorylase deficiencies are not disproven but are less likely than type 1 glycogen storage disease.

THERAPEUTIC: The patient was treated with a regular diet in the hospital, and at no time demonstrated evidence of hypoglycemia. On discharge he was given a special nonlactose containing formula, and a diet free of galactose, sucrose and fructose.

DISCUSSION: Flat blood glucose curve with administration of glucagon, after priming the liver with galactose, suggests either glucose-6-phosphatase deficiency or phosphorylase deficiency, e.g., glycogen storage disease, type 1 or type 6.

PROBLEM #4. RIGHT HYDROCELE

PROBLEM #5. RIGHT UPPER LOBE PNEUMONIA

SUBJECTIVE: Cough and irritability.

OBJECTIVE: Chest X ray on 4/22 showed a right lower lobe and minimal left lower lobe pneumonia; the sputum grew Homophilus influenzae. Chest X ray on the day of discharge showed marked clearing of the infiltrates.

THERAPEUTIC: Ampicillin for 7 days.

PROBLEM #6. DRUG ERUPTION

SUBJECTIVE: On the day prior to discharge, the patient developed a rash.

OBJECTIVE: Symmetrically involving the anterior and posterior surfaces of the trunk were nonconfluent, erythematous macules. These seemed to to pruritic. On the day of discharge, a rash had become confluent on the trunk, face, and back; the macular rash had spread to the extremities. A dermatological consultant agreed with the diagnosis of drug eruption, probably secondary to ampicillin.

THERAPEUTIC: Ampicillin was stopped and Benadryl at 5 mg/kg/day was instituted.

3rd CMGH ADMISSION, May 2, 1968.

PROBLEM #7. FEVER AND VOMITING

SUBJECTIVE: Fever beginning about 12 hours after discharge. Vomited 2 feedings the night prior to admission, then retained 2 feedings. Twelve hours prior to admission had generalized seizure and brought to EW [emergency ward]. Continued vomiting of glucose water at home and admitted.

Resolution of vomiting with glucose water in 1st 36 hours of hospitalization.

OBJECTIVE: EW: LP [lumbar puncture] negative, glucose and protein not obtained. Dextrostix 40 mg%. Cultures of CSF [cerebral spinal fluid], blood, urine, throat, normal or sterile.

THERAPEUTIC: 1. Glucose water
2. Similac
3. 3200-H (nonlactose containing formula)

PROBLEM #3. GLYCOGEN STORAGE DISEASE

SUBJECTIVE: Seizure (see #7); this did not recur.

OBJECTIVE: Physical examination showed liver edge 7–9 cm below right costal margin; otherwise unchanged from 2nd admission.

HCT 28–31%; MCV 87, MCH 31, MCHC 35.

Blood glucose was determined on three consecutive occasions, four hours after feeding of 3200-H; values were: 19.3 mg%, 58.1, 74.1.

WBC [white blood cell] stain with toluidine blue showed no metachromatic granules; EEG, EKG normal. Neurologist felt seizure most likely due to hypoglycemia.

THERAPEUTIC: 1. Diet as for 2nd admission
2. Formula 3200-H.

D. Starbuck, M.D.

APPENDIX D

Pediatric Problem Sheet

The following format is an adaptation of the ordinary problem list to serve the special requirements of a pediatric service.

ACTIVE PROBLEMS	INACTIVE PROBLEMS

#1. Well child care
  a. Family history*
  b. Child rearing†
  c. Development‡
  d. Immunizations§

#2.

#3.

. . . .

In pediatrics, in addition to the usual data base obtained for the adult, pregnancy and birth history should be included and special

---

* Elements of the family history (tuberculosis or sickle-cell disease in a parent) that bear upon the health of the child. Where medical problems related to the family history occur in the child, they should of course be separately listed.

† Toilet training, diet, etc.

‡ Using standard flow sheets: Colorado Intrauterine Growth Charts, Children's Medical Center Anthropometric Chart, Denver Developmental Screening Test, etc.

§ Using standard forms.

questionnaires for given age groups are necessary. Selected elements of the physical examination, moreover, should be performed regularly during development.

A Case History of an
Ambulatory Patient
with Multiple Problems

Problem List:

   #1. Rheumatic Heart Disease: 10/28/68

   H/O Rheumatic Fever age 22—hospitalization (see
   summary)

   Monthly penicillin prophylaxis

   (Rheumatic heart disease—valvular—unspecified, class
   I A)

   #2. Diabetes Mellitus: 10/28/68

   Poorly controlled

   Gestational diabetes—10 yrs ago

   Symptomatic non-ketotic Dx at . . . 2 yrs ago (see
   report)

   #3. Essential Vascular Hypertension: 10/28/68

   H/O Preeclampsia

   Borderline renal function

#4. Chronic Hoarseness: 10/28/68

Thickening of L vocal cord

#5. Recent Resolving URI with pharyngitis: 10/28/68

#6. Anxiety Secondary to: (with depression) 11/13/68

a. Delinquent behavior of adolescent daughter, K.
b. Marital problems: husband in prison
c. Physical problems involving her own and children's health

#7. H/O Syncopal Episodes X 2: 11/13/68

Associated FH of convulsive disorder (daughter K.)

#8. H/O Chronic P.I.D. with recurrent subacute exacerbations:

(see . . . OPD notes)

#9. Irregular Menses: 11/13/68

Menorrhagia, metrorrhagia
Minimally enlarged uterus

History and physical examination and initial lab work (the data base) and the initial plan were recorded in the usual manner and will be omitted in the presentation of this particular case. The emphasis here is on the titled, numbered progress notes as they should be used in ambulatory care for patients with multiple medical, social, and psychiatric problems.

11/13/68 *#1. Rheumatic Heart Disease:*

Bicillin. Due today to Mrs. B. See history.

#2. Diabetes Mellitus: (See flow chart)

Subj: Polyuria, polydipsia and appetite continue unabated. Has no vaginal pruritis. Pt. has never been on any hypoglycemic Rx.

Obj: See flow chart.

Plan: Start Phenformin—T.D. o/o50 q day.

> *Interpretation:* Uncontrolled diabetes although not severely symptomatic. I hope for the benefit of the anorexogenic effect of Phenformin. The pt's. present anxiety is undoubtedly contributing to compulsive eating as well as poor control.
>
> We await CMGH records.

#3. H/O Hypertension:

Subj: None at present. Has been on Naqua & Reserpine intermittently and low salt.

Obj: See flow chart. Normotensive today.

Plan: Careful evaluation of renal function after P.E. done. I.V.P.'s—WNL (11/27/68).

> 2 hrs. Creatinine clearance—(25,65 cc'min Clearance #1, #2.)(?)
>
> Repeat urine on an aglycosuric spec. (1.045, 1.035 c̄ CHO)

#6. Anxiety: 2° to psychosocial problems.

> a) Delinquent behavior of teen-age daughter—16 yr old who has been followed in the seizure clinic at CMGH for years, is now off anti-convulsants—apparently because of no documentation by LP or EEG of convulsive disorder—has been truant from school and has run away from home—3 weeks recently—followed by Detention Home care for a week. She has been discharged from seizure clinic.
>
> b) Recent divorce from husband who is "an habitual criminal" and is presently in jail. Her daughter is

very devoted to her father and the mother has not told her about the divorce. The father will be released from jail in one month and the parent is very apprehensive about the daughter when this occurs.

Plan: Enroll daughter for medical care. Get CMGH records on daughter.

Immediate referral to Mental Health Unit and contact c̄ Miss R. L. at the "Youth Center" on ——— Rd. who has been counseling this girl.

#4. Chronic Hoarseness:

Since indirect laryngoscopy is negative, will simply follow. Chronic sinusitis may contribute some to Sx —perhaps psychogenic component.

ENT referral may eventually be planned if Sx continue to be a problem.

11/21/68 144/100 P:60 (See flow chart)

12/13/68 T:98.02r   Wt: 161

#1. Rheumatic Heart Disease: Nurse's Notes.

1.2 million units Penicillin (BiCillin) IM today for RF prophylaxis.

12/27/68   #6. Anxiety: Secondary to psychosocial problems.

Initially resistant to seeing me because "I'm not crazy." Did accept talking about her daughter and then talked about herself. Daughter has apparently been less of a problem to her over last month and is considering attending work-study program. Mrs. W. is continuing to have insomnia and "losing control" of her arm. This latter could be on an hysterical basis, but this will be checked with Dr. W. to rule out physical etiology. Mrs. W. wants help and is willing to see me re her anxiety as long as we also recognize and offer support re her daughter's behavior.

Question: Would her daughter's behavior be related to sub-clinical seizure equivalents?

Psychologist's Note.

1/3/69 *#6. Anxiety*: Secondary to family psychosocial problem.

> Telephone call to Mrs. L. at Youth Service indicates that she is seeing *both* Mrs. W. and her daughter weekly for counseling. Therefore, I feel that we should not get involved directly with this problem with Mrs. W., but let the Youth Service counselor handle it. If the problem persists after Youth Service completes the counseling, a new referral may be appropriate. Mrs. L. will notify of any change in status of their contact.
>
> Psychologist's Note.

1/9/69 Failed Appt.

1/15/69 *#1*. T: 98° Wt: 167½

> *#6. Anxiety*: Family problems: Dr. L. will review pediatric charts and assign them to pediatricians.
>
> > *K.*—age 16—daughter
> > Already enrolled here.
> > Has a physician assigned (LBW).
> > Adolescent depression & delinquency.
> >
> > *V.*—age 10—daughter
> > Registered but not assigned.
> > Has a heart murmur.
> >
> > *S.*—age 7—daughter
> > Adenoids & tonsils.
> > Registered but not assigned.
> > Allergies.
> >
> > *T.*—age 5—daughter
> > Anemic, has nosebleeds.
> > Registered but not assigned.
> >
> > *P.*—age 3½—daughter
> > "Stomach disorder"—has been seen daily in Well Clinic.

#4. Chronic Hoarseness:

Subj: Worse today.

Obj. (See ENT consult note 1/6/68) "Thickening of left vocal cord."

Plan: Recommendation of ENT consult discussed in detail with the patient.

↑ humidification; and voice rest.

↓ smoking:

#2. Diabetes Mellitus:

Subj: Nocturia 4–5 X.
Is not clear whether insomnia or nocturia comes first.

Obj: Control is poor (see flow chart & home diary record).

Rx: Add Orinase 0/5 bid. Continue Phenformin 0/050 P.P. sugar, today.

#3. Essential Hypertension:

Subj: Headaches related to emotional crises which she tends to attribute to blood pressure.

Obj: B.P. 152/110.
No edema.

Rx: Continue Hydrodiuril
0/050 q day.
1000 mg Na.
Review diet next visit.
Get CO_2 ⎫
    K ⎬ next visit.

#7. H/O Syncope X2:

Subj: Per Dr. C, this history was reviewed today.
Two episodes: both associated c̄ intense emotional upset.
One occurred while pt. under observation for ? pelvic surgery.

Associated—but separate Sx—coarse intention trem-
or of Rt. hand when pt. is nervous or upset. Relieved by Meprobamate.

Now—infrequent, or none at all.

Obj: No new findings on review of neurological exam.

Plan: Consider EEG after receiving CMGH information
on K's convulsive disorder.
Ret. 2/20/69.
See family record.

2/18/69 #2. *Diabetes Mellitus*: (see flow chart) T:98 Wt: 170

Control is poor.
Phenformin-TD 0/050 bid.
Orinase 0/5 bid.
1200 calorie—low salt diet reviewed c̄ patient.

#3. *Essential Hypertension:*

See diabetes—hypertension flow chart.
Continue Hydrodiuril 0/050 q day.
Review of salt restriction.

#4. *Chronic Hoarseness:*

Sx: Worse symptomatically.
Has another 10 days of Tetracycline (250 tid. Rx'd
by U.H. ENT Consult).

Rx: Pt. urged to complete Rx of antibiotic.
Voice rest.
No smoking (now 2 pks.) before reaching any con-
clusions.
To keep appointment at ENT.

#6. *Anxiety:*

Sx: Worse today—pt. preoccupied c̄ somatic Sx and
complains of "failing memory."

Rx: Continue Librium o/o1o tid.

Continue sessions with daughter's Youth Center counselor.

FU visit to Mental Health Unit.

RTC in one month.

3/24/69 *#1. Rheumatic Heart Disease*: T: 98.6 P: 79 R: 18 Wt: 170

BiCillin 1.2 M units IM today.

#4. Chronic Hoarseness:

Admission to ENT surgery at Univ. Hospitals scheduled. April 7 (with Dr. W.)—for direct laryngoscopy.

#1. Rheumatic Heart Disease:

Sx: Fleeting substernal chest pains and migratory arthralgia; minor Sx in shoulders, knees without objective signs.

No ↑ dyspnea.

Wt. has not changed.

Obj: Joints neg.

Lung bases clear.

Heart: ii/vi soft blowing basal M as before. Not enl.

Extremities: no edema.

Classify as R.H.D. Valvular, unspecified—functional 1-A.

Rx: Continue prophylactic I.M.

BiCillin as per monthly schedule.

#2. Diabetes Mellitus:

Sx: Continues to have nocturia X 4–6. No dysuria.

Considerable incontinence c̄ coughing.

Poor dietary control.

Obj: 3+ → 4+ glycosuria most of the time.

Rx: ↑ Phenformin T.D. to bid.
 ↑   Tolbutamide 1/o ——— 1/o.
      Obtain: CO_2 K
              Bun
              Bilirubin
              Alk phosph.
              Post-prandial
              CHO (random)
              Hct, Hgb.
              WBC
              Sed rate
              ASO

#3. Essential Hypertension:

Subj: No special Symp. Headaches continue, which patient tends to attribute to high B.P.

Obj: B.P.: 158/104.

Rx: Hydrodiuril o/o50 q day.
     CO_2 K.
     Uric acid.

#4. Chronic Hoarseness:

Sx: No sore throat. But hoarseness is constant and quite severe—difficult to evaluate psychic component: patient says headaches ↑ with fatigue, nerves.
Is scheduled for ENT admission on April 7 but we have not been informed of this nor of what surgical procedure is planned. Pt. states that U.H. ENT Consult does not know her medical complications although they were outlined in her records to them.

Plan: Call in to Dr. W.—ENT Resident, to discuss the situation.

#6. Chronic Anxiety:

Sx: Continues to worry about malignancy. Feels depressed. In the face of all of these problems is nevertheless contemplating marriage, in the near future! Also plans to become employed!

A number of agencies besides ourselves have suddenly become involved in planning for psychiatric help including a Glenville agency, referral to U.H., to H. Pavillion, and our Mental Health Unit as well as the Youth Center (Miss L.).

Dr. C. has been notified.

3/28/69   *Screening Nurse's Notes:*

Anxious female c̄ complaint of frontal headache since Monday.

Pain began while pt. was waiting at hospital for daughter to be admitted for T & A. T—98. Pt. is very upset about her own scheduled admission to U.H. next week.

B.P. 192/? (Palpation).

R.N.

#6. *Anxiety:*

Sx: Pt. came in a walk-in basis because of severe headache, anxiety depression. A number of associated events are related:

daughter's scheduled admission for T & A on Monday was cancelled because of no space. Pt. having extreme anxiety over her own ENT admission for a direct laryngoscopy on April 7 and her fears of laryngeal cancer. She is also associating this with fantasies about her mother's death at 48 of heart disease 12 yrs ago, and her father's death at 52, and her baby's death of strangulation. Severe headache is *not* a usual expression of anxiety for her, she says.

Obj: B.P.: 200/128   P: 88

Pt. weeping, dishevelled and depressed.

Fundi—pupils miotic so poorly visualized. Discs flat. No H. or E. (hemorrhages or exudates).

Chest—clear

Neurological—neg.

Rx: Reassurance c̄ respect to statistical chances of malignancy of larynx.

Review of grief and depression over losses dating back to more than 12 years ago and their association with her present fears for her own declining physical and mental health.

Librium o/o1o bid→ qid, to include an HS dose.

#8. Headaches (New Sx):

Sx: Patient has had intense orbital and frontal pain since Monday (5 days). Onset in waiting room at U.H. to admit daughter for T & A. (She also overheard my telephone conversation c̄ Dr. W.—ENT consultant re her own operation.) With her many psychiatric Sx she has never had severe headaches, before now.

Obj: B.P. markedly over previous levels—200/128.
No other new findings.
Fundi O.K. (See note on hypertension)
Neurol. normal.

Rx: Continue Hydrodiuril.
o/o50 bid.
Start Hydralazine o/o1o qid for the next few days. When we see her Wednesday, consider increase to o/o25 qid.
(I would be fearful of reserpine in this pt. because of her depression.)

> *Discussion:* It is difficult to assess the sudden onset of headaches with pt. because of: ↑ intensity of anxieties over personal problems, and because of the ↑ B.P., which is marked and reason for concern.

4/1/69 *#6. Anxiety:*

Seen today on request of Dr. W. because of exacerbation of anxiety 2° to upcoming surgical procedure. Was less depressed today and able to discuss her reaction to ENT consult. Has a great fear re possible malignancy. However, she also relates her depression to recent celebration of deceased mother's birthday. She apparently gets a card each year and writes appropriate sentiments in it, then displays it on mantel. She recognizes the inappropriateness of the prolonged grief, but confesses she is powerless to stop it. She is looking forward to her marriage and it sounds as if he would be a good man for her. She states that the only problem will be to control her "bossiness." We discussed all these things and I reassured her again re the scheduled procedure. She seems calmer and able to cooperate at this point. I told her to call me if she gets more nervous toward the end of the week.

Recommendation: The procedure should be thoroughly explained to her and more reassurance given. In addition the results must be carefully interpreted to her because she will misinterpret them if they are presented vaguely.

Dr. C.

4/2/69   *#3. Hypertension:* (See flow chart)

BP: 144/110   T: 98.6   Wt: 169½

Sx: Marked improvement in headache, dizziness as well as anxiety.

Obj: BP ↓ .
No edema.

Discussion: Obviously impossible to sort out contribution to improvement to difference in supportive psycho. Rx and reassurance, and/or addition of Hydralazine to Rx regimen. Since patient has probable borderline renal function, she will bear close following.

Plan: ↑ Hydralazine o/025 tid.
Continue Hydrodiuril o/050 bid.
Librium o/010 tid.

#2. Diabetes Mellitus:

Sx: ↓ nocturia o–2 times (less than before) despite D/C Phenformin.

Blood sugar drawn last week not yet reported.
4+/0 /0 in today's urine. Home diary continues to
show 2+→ 3+ glycosuria.

Rx: Continue Tolbutamide 1/0 - 0/5 - 1/0 daily.

#*1. Rheumatic Heart Disease:*
Next BiCillin due 4/22/69.

#*6. Anxiety:*

Sx: Much improvement c̄ reassurance of Dr. C.'s interview, and last week's visit here, lessening of depression.

Obj: Patient calm and quiet, not crying today.

Rx: Continue 0/010 Librium tid. and HS only.
Follow through on ENT admission for laryngoscopy.

ABBREVIATIONS:

H/O	= history of ...
L	= left
URI	= upper respiratory infection
FH	= family history
P.I.D.	= pelvic inflammatory disease
WNL	= within normal limits
I.V.P.'s	= intravenous pyelograms
CHO	= carbohydrate
Sx	= symptoms
ENT	= Ear, Nose, Throat
FU	= follow-up
RTC	= Return to Clinic
R.H.D.	= Rheumatic Heart Disease
HS	= bed-time

Preparing and Maintaining the Problem-Oriented Record:
The PROMIS Method *

I have devoted watchful attention to the use of the "Modulor" and to the supervision of its use. Sometimes I have seen on the drawing board designs that were displeasing, badly put together: "But it was one with a Modulor." Well then, forget about the Modulor. Do you imagine that the Modulor is a panacea for clumsiness or carelessness? Scrap it. If all you can do with a Modulor is to produce such horrors as these, drop it. Your eyes are your judge, the only one you should know. Judge with your eyes, gentlemen. Let us repeat together again in simple good faith, that the Modulor is a working tool, a precision instrument: a keyboard shall we say, a piano, a tuned piano. The piano has been tuned; it is up to you to play it well. The Modulor does not confer talent, still less genius. It does not make the dull subtle; it only offers them the facility of a sure measure. But out of the unlimited choices of combinations of the Modulor, the choice is yours.

The Modulor is but a simple tool for speeding things up, for getting across the pot holes and puddles in the way of progress. The real objective of the technicians of design is to compose, create, invent, find, show what they have up their sleeve, create proportion. The Modulor, a working tool, sweeps the track clean: it is you, not it, who are the runners! There is the answer in a nutshell

---

*This section was developed with the assistance of Stephen Schacher, M.D., at the PROMIS Laboratory.

for you. It is you who has got to do the running. Some people are always wanting to buy from the chemist, or the seller of dreams, a little gadget for making talent or genius. Poor fools! Nothing exists except what is deep within us, and the Modulor only does the housework—no more. Which is a great deal!

Le Corbusier, *The Modulor*

The problem-oriented medical record consists of four phases of medical activity:

1. Establishment of a data base.
2. Formulation of a list of all problems.
3. The initial plans for each problem.
4. Progress notes on each problem.

ESTABLISHMENT OF A DATA BASE

The data base is the initial collection of information about the patient.

At the present time the size of the data base is a private matter for most physicians in this country. Some physicians may ask five allergy questions, some ask fifty-five. Some routinely look at the patient's joints; others, unless he has symptoms, never do. Some sigmoidoscope the patient at regular intervals to look for cancer or other disturbances; for others, this is not routine.

It is also apparent that the size of the data base collected on any individual patient varies with the nature of his complaint. Individuals receiving episodic care may have a very small data base collected, while patients with multiple or complicated problems may have a very extensive one.

But, whether the data base is small or large, there is currently no way of knowing, by looking at a physician's medical record, precisely what is included in the data base. That is, there is no way of deciding if information is omitted from the record because it was considered to be irrelevant, or merely because it was never obtained.

The point here is neither that all physicians should ask the same standard questions nor is it that a big data base is better than a small one. Rather, the important thing is that the data base be specified precisely, so that it is clear from looking at the medical record which questions were asked and which were not, what part of the physical examination was performed and what was omitted, and so on. Without this there can be no effective quality control (audit) in medical practice, and each physician is left to create his own standard.

The following pages describe the data base presented in *Medical Records, Medical Education, and Patient Care*.

The data base consists of six basic elements:

1. Chief complaint
2. Patient profile
3. Present illness or illnesses
4. Past history and systems review
5. Physical examination
6. Baseline laboratory examination

1. *Chief complaint.* The chief complaint should be a concise statement of the reason the patient seeks medical attention, preferably in the patient's own words.

2. *Patient profile.* This should be an explicit account of how the patient spends his routine day. It should not be limited to the familiar insensitive "social history" (2 packs a day, moderate drinking, born in Alabama). Rather, it should contain information which allows the physician to plan realistically and sympathetically for the practical welfare of the patient. It is composed of information obtained from the patient or other informants and does not include conclusions or observations made by the physician.

Example: General: Who is the patient; what is his environment?

Life style: What are his eating, sleeping, work, and recreational habits? How does he spend the day?

Family unit: Who is in the family; what relationships exist?

Housing unit, work environment etc.

The above is not a suggested format, but an illustration of the kinds of information to be included.

3. *Present illness or illnesses.* Present illnesses fall roughly into 2 categories:

Those in which the problem is undiagnosed and begins with a complaint or an abnormal finding. The statement should begin with an appropriate title such as "abdominal pain," and the history should then be recorded chronologically.

Those that result from relapses in already well-established disorders such as rheumatic heart disease or myocardial infarction with heart failure, diabetes, and peripheral vascular disease. The paragraph should be titled with the disease process itself.

In both categories the statement consists of:

Symptomatic information (e.g., details concerning pain)
Objective information (e.g., a gastrointestinal series from an old record or data from another hospital)
(Information concerning previous treatment and significant negatives should be included under "symptomatic" if obtained from the patient, and under "objective" if obtained from a record.)

These two types of information (symptomatic and objective) should be recorded *separately* and not interwoven in a single chronological sequence. If relationships are important among many variables over a span of time, then a flowsheet should be constructed. Interrelationships are either completely obscure in narrative data or only partially seen. Because of this, false cause-and-effect relationships may be deduced.

Problems unrelated to each other and problems requiring separate management should be discussed separately. All available relevant information should be presented. If particular information is of doubtful reliability, such doubts should be expressed or the information omitted.

4. *Past history and systems review.* The past history and systems review should be based on a series of explicit and logically arranged questions in a branching pattern. The questions should

either be arranged on a printed questionnaire, or as in the PROMIS Laboratory, be an integral part of the computer system. Individuals unfamiliar with this history should ask to be shown copies of a printed questionnaire or, if possible, perform part of the history in the computer on themselves.

The review of systems used in the PROMIS Laboratory appears in Appendix A of this book. It was created by asking specialists in the appropriate areas to define a set of questions which they considered to be an adequate systems review. Though it has been found to be useful in practice in its current form, especially in its definition of a precise set of questions which are always asked, we are no longer satisfied with it. In subsequent editions of this book it will be replaced by a new systems review. The reason why it is no longer satisfactory is that it is not based on a metastructure. That is, there is no underlying structure which allows the user to predict from looking at one system what the questions in the other systems will be like. As a result the quality and completeness of any individual section cannot be assessed.

The systems review which will appear in subsequent editions of this book will be based on the following metastructure:

A. *Current Function:* What is the current level of function of the system under consideration? When abnormalities are detected, we will ask, "Have they been previously evaluated?"

i. If they have been evaluated, what are the results, and what is the patient's attitude about this evaluation and treatment?

ii. If a functional abnormality has not previously been evaluated a more detailed history is required. It is at this point that the systems review and the record of the present illness overlap. In the systems review enough easily answered questions should be asked of the patient to alert the physician to the presence of a problem. Full problem descriptions can then be obtained by the physician and should appear in the record of the present illness.

B. *Past Function:* What functional abnormalities previously existed but have now disappeared? If there were such abnormalities, what was done and what is the patient's attitude about it?

C. *Future Function:* What demographic data are available to indicate the amount and types of future risk to the patient, and is he aware of these (for example, smoking, seat belts, diet)? What preventative measures does he follow (e.g., exercise)?

Our experience with computerization has repeatedly emphasized the value of a metastructure, and our failure to employ one in the systems review is now being corrected.

5. *Physical examination.* It is difficult to deal in detail with the physical examination in this outline. A few general guidelines, however, should be restated:

The examination should be thorough and accurate.

Significant portions of the examination should not be omitted at the whim of the examiner.

If a paper record is being used, it should be clear precisely what was examined and what was not. Entries such as "Eyes: normal" only make sense if a pre-printed sheet is available on which the specific parts of the examination routinely performed are recorded.

If a computerized record is used, as in the PROMIS Laboratory, the guidelines built into the system will make clear what is performed and what is omitted.

6. *Baseline laboratory examination.* Baseline laboratory examinations will undoubtedly vary from one medical center to another and among different population groups, age groups, and geographic areas. The essential point, though, is that it matters less what tests are included than that it be precisely stated in the record what tests are being routinely ordered.

THE PROBLEM LIST

The first page of the patient's record should consist of a numbered problem list. It is a "table of contents" and an "index" combined, and the care with which it is constructed determines the quality of the whole record. Inherent in the problem-oriented approach to data organization in the medical record is the necessity for completeness in the formulation of the problem list. The precision with which plans are formulated and followed through is directly related to the precision and integrity with which the problems are initially defined.

The student or physician should list *all* the patient's problems, past as well as present, social and psychiatric as well as medical. The list should not contain diagnostic guesses. It should simply state the problems at a level of refinement consistent with the physician's understanding, running the gamut from precise diagnosis to the isolated, unexplained finding.

If a beginner enters cardiomegaly, edema, hepatomegaly, and shortness of breath as four separate problems, he thereby emphatically admits that he does not recognize cardiac failure when he sees it. But the important point is that nothing is lost. On the contrary, the interest of more experienced observers is immediately aroused, the patient's problems are combined as is appropriate under a single heading on the original list, and the student has learned something. The system does not prevent analysis and integration. It merely reveals the extent to which they are performed and defines the level of sophistication at which the physician functions.

The problem list should contain ALL the patient's problems classified as follows:

A. Problems classified by field of interest and level of understanding.

   1. Medical problems, classified as one of the following:

      a. A diagnosis (e.g., arteriosclerotic heart disease, followed by the principal manifestation that requires management, as heart failure).

         i. Guesses and questionable or probable diagnoses and "rule outs" are *not* included here but are put in the *initial plan.*

         ii. If a given diagnosis has several major manifestations, each of which requires individual management and separate progress notes, the second manifestation is presented as a second problem and designated as secondary to the major diagnosis.

Example: Problem No. 1. ASHD with heart failure.
Problem No. 2. Supraventricular tachycardia—2° to Problem No. 1.
If the several manifestations do not require individual management, they can follow the diagnosis.

Example: Problem No. 1. Cirrhosis manifested by jaundice and ascites (minimal).

    b. A physiologic finding (e.g., heart failure), followed by either the phrase "etiology unknown" or "2° to a diagnosis" (e.g., ASHD).

    c. A symptom or a physical finding (e.g., dyspnea).

    d. An abnormal laboratory finding (e.g., abnormal EKG).

2. Social problems (e.g., bankruptcy, severe delinquency).

3. Demographic problems (i.e., regarding health hazards; e.g., smoking, seat belts, alcohol, hunting safety).

4. Psychiatric problems (described in non-technical language, if physician is unfamiliar with sophisticated psychiatric terminology).

B. Problems classified by status

1. Active problems

If the physician's time is limited, or the patient's condition prevents the acquisition of a complete data base, or if previous charts and records have not been completely reviewed, then problem No. 1 should always be "incomplete data base." The omitted items should be noted as: "Incomplete Data Base, pelvic exam omitted." By noting an incomplete data base as problem No. 1, the physician is continually reminded that he may be dealing with a problem out of context. (E.g., anticoagulation being given for embolism without the knowledge that an ulcer or bleeding diathesis may be present.)

2. Inactive or resolved problems, including any previously significant difficulty which might recur or lead to complications.

The problem list should be modified in the following manner; *all changes should be dated:*

24 hours should be allowed for reformulation of the initial problem list if necessary. This interval enables attending physicians, chief residents, and consultants to help define the problems. The reformulated list should not be destroyed, only modified.

A problem should be modified by inserting an arrow, followed by the new diagnosis, or by "dropped" or "resolved."

When several problems turn out to be separate manifestations of a single problem (such as pericarditis and arthritis becoming lupus), then the two may be grouped together and designated as lupus, using the number and position of the *first* of the two problems. The unused number then becomes inactive for all subsequent visits.

When a new problem appears, it should be added to the list.

Minor episodes may be titled "temporary problems" in the *progress notes.* When a second progress note is written, it will be easy to decide if it should be transferred to the problem list or dropped.

The numbered' problem list should be the first page of the patient record and should be enlarged and displayed like an X ray at surgery.

Consultant notes should be treated as follows:
The consultant should state the number and title of the problem for which he was consulted.

He should state his general conclusion about the problem. For example, indicate agreement or restate the problem as now understood ("#2, cirrhosis" should be revised to "chronic active hepatitis," for there is no proof of actual hepatic fibrosis or its consequences).

He should state the major recommendation for resolving the problem.

He should include any new additions to the four elements of the problem:

subjective—new data only
objective—new data only
assessment—consultant's opinions, concerns, and reference sources
plan—specific recommendations, in outline, for data collection, problem formulation, and monitoring or measuring progress

The consultant should review the total problem list. If, as a result of his examination of the patient, he has uncovered new problems or has revisions to make on established problems, he should do so by writing numbered, titled progress notes under the appropriate problem.

THE INITIAL PLAN

Plans for the possible diagnosis and management of each problem, keyed by number to the problem list, should be prepared as the next logical step after the problem list has been formulated. *Each problem should have its own plan, numbered correspondingly,* so that an experienced observer can see at a glance whether an anemia, or a urinary tract infection, for example, has a complete and reasonable plan. Too many serious omissions occur when sleeping pills, laboratory studies, diet, and side rails are all mixed up as the physician writes the order sheet in a haphazard fashion.

When a well-conceived plan is written at the outset, all that is necessary for long periods of time in the progress notes is a record of the data as they are produced. The initial statement of plans is important because it establishes the character of the further data that are to be obtained and the treatment that is to be given.

The patient profile and complete list of problems should be reexamined before plans are made for any problem. Awareness of the patient's way of life and of the whole range of his problems is essential in the avoidance of surgical and medical treatments that may be disastrous in a given context, though they are indicated for a particular problem in isolation.

Through a more thorough awareness of the patient's milieu, the physician is in a better position to help him establish or modify personal objectives, with regard, for instance, to returning to work, caring for children, or entering a nursing home.

Many physicians are inclined to believe it unnecessary to plan specifically the education of the patient, but this seriously neglected aspect of patient care is an integral part of the initial plan. It is naive to expect that when patients are discharged they will understand and manage their own procedures, drugs, and diets, especially when that information is improvised by the physician at the moment of discharge.

Furthermore, patient education should not only be directed at therapeutic directions, but should also include a whole range of information about the problems. Only a carefully prepared problem-oriented record will avoid the risk of omitting discussion of any problems.

As a doctor learns best through his own work and his own progress notes, if led by the data and carefully observed by his peers, so does a patient learn best from his own experiences, when led by the data on his own problems and carefully guided by his physician.

In the last analysis, the patient with chronic disease must in large part be his own physician. If he does not understand his own illness and treament, moments of reprimand and irritability in the office or clinic will provide little in the way of correctives. It is not surprising that studies of compliance in medical therapy indicate a level of non-compliance of 25–50%.

Each problem should have its own plans, numbered correspondingly to the problem list:

A. Plans for the *collection* of further data in order to establish a diagnosis or facilitate management.

> To "rule out" is a *diagnostic plan*. The explicit manner in which the "rule out" is to be done should be clearly

delineated, as to which tests will be performed and in what order. For each test, it should be stated what the pre-conditions of the test are, and what result will be accepted as sufficient evidence for the rule-out.

For example, hypertension, rule out aldosteronism.

Pre-condition: (Level of salt in diet defined.)

Test acceptance: (Value of K^+ which will be accepted as ruling out this diagnosis should be stated.)

By carefully stating the rule-out plan in this manner and reviewing it before tests are performed, the need to repeat poorly performed tests will be markedly reduced.

A plan for ruling out certain diagnoses should also take into consideration economic factors. A single day in any hospital is extremely expensive compared to most individual tests. All those tests which can be reasonably performed on the same day (in *parallel*) should be specified. Those tests which should only be done after the results of previous tests are known (in *series*) should be described in the order they will be done.

When tests are to be done in series, the logic involved should be clearly defined so that anyone looking at the plan will know which tests should be done next, when the day's test results are returned to the ward.

When further information is required for skillful management of a problem, general statements should be avoided and specific parameters to be followed in a progress note or on a flowsheet should be identified instead. There should be an indication of the frequency with which they should be obtained.

B. Plans for *treatment* with specific procedures or drugs. Entries such as "postural drainage" or "fluids" are not specific enough.

C. Plans for *education* of the patient about his illness and his part in managing it.

PROGRESS NOTES

The progress notes should be written in a form which relates them clearly and unmistakably to the problem. Each note should be preceded by the number and title of the appropriate problem, so that the reader knows, for instance, that it is the progress of the anemia (or the urinary tract infection) which is under discussion.

If a new problem is being discussed, it should be added to the original list, and dated and numbered accordingly. No progress note should be written without attention being paid to previous progress notes on the same problem.

Progress notes are the most crucial part of the medical record. Whereas faulty understanding and defective decision-making may be expected at the outset of a new case, failure to follow up rigorously the results of those decisions is inexcusable. Action without follow-up is arrogance, especially where the objects of that action are living systems about which nothing is completely understood and in which conditions never remain fixed. Naturally, to be intelligible may mean to be found out, but it is this explicitness that leads to sound education and sound medical care.

Progress notes provide the *feedback* on the problem list and the plans. As has often been said, any system without a feedback loop runs wild. By not structuring progress notes and relating them to the appropriate problem and plan, the traditional medical record has become a system without feedback.

Failure to recognize the progress note as the most important part of the record nullifies the most basic attitude of science and of research, for it is only through careful observation of results that new questions can be asked, new plans formulated, sloppy thinking exposed, and clearer understanding achieved. In other words, the physician should be part of a sophisticated guidance system with corrective feedback loops, not an oracle that knows answers.

Each note should be preceded by the number and title of the appropriate problem. Nurses' notes, social service notes, and physical medicine notes should *not* be separate parts of the medical record, but should themselves be progress notes of the types recommended here.

Problem statements include the following:

(S) Subjective data: (e.g., qualitative and quantitative description of the symptoms *appropriate* to the problem) .

(O) Objective data: (e.g., actual clinical findings, X-ray results, or laboratory findings *appropriate* to the problem, preferably in the order and context designated in the original plan) .

(A) Assessment: this portion of the progress note should deal directly with the subjective and objective portions of the note. If the problem statement, subjective data, and objective data are *all* internally consistent, then little needs to be said in this section. Implicit in a detailed plan is what one must be thinking.

  However, if symptomatic data are not consistent with objective data, or neither are consistent with statement of the problem or the plan, then an assessment of this state of affairs is indicated. Significant internal inconsistencies between symptomatic and objective data should lead one to *question the accuracy of the statement* of the original problem. Herein lies the feedback loop, without which the medical record as a system runs wild.

(P) Plan: departures from the original well thought-out plan and contingency actions should obviously be made when indicated by circumstances that could not have been foreseen—but random, poorly thought-out plunges into procedures and drugs are to be avoided.

Regarding resident notes:

The conventional extended resident note is not recommended.

After working up the patient, the resident should review and correct the intern's problem list by inserting "agree" or a specific amendment after each problem.

The resident should insist that the list of problems be complete and current, and that the level of resolution of each problem be apparent.

If an intern fails to develop under a given resident, documentation of this failure, explicit in the medical record and particularly in the resident's notes, should be made available to the faculty, preferably by the resident himself.

Regarding operative notes:

These should appear as numbered and titled progress notes on the appropriate problem.

If operative findings are diagnostic, the problem list should be modified accordingly.

Additional useful information from surgery should be stated under the appropriate problem number.

Complications following surgery should be stated as new problems followed by the entry "secondary to problem No. [the original problem]."

The following objections and questions are the ones visitors most commonly ask when visiting the PROMIS Laboratory.

1. The problem list frequently results in fragmentation of diagnostic entries.

   Ans: As has already been stated in the text, if a complete analysis is done on each finding, integration of related findings occurs with clarity and inevitability. Failure to integrate findings into a valid single entity can almost always be traced to incomplete understanding of all the implications of one or all of them. If a beginner enters cardiomegaly, edema, shortness of breath, and heptatomegaly as four separate problems, he thereby emphatically admits that he does not recognize cardiac failure when he sees it. But the important point is that nothing is lost. On the contrary, the interest of more experienced observers is aroused, the patient's problems are combined as is appropriate under a single heading on the original list, and they are carried one step closer to diagnosis and treatment. The system does not prevent analysis and integration; it merely reveals the extent to which they are performed and defines the level of sophistication at which the physician functions.

But the question that really needs to be asked is *not* whether the problem-oriented record results in fragmentation of diagnosis, but whether the problem-oriented record *can help prevent the fragmentation of patient care that has resulted from dealing with patients' problems out of the context of a total problem list.* For it must be remembered that patients do not specialize. And the answer to this question is that this is precisely what the problem-oriented record has been designed to do.

2. It would take forever to list all the problems on some patients.

Ans: There are, of course, many patients with complaints about every part of their body. For this reason, there is included in the computer system a problem titled "multiple somatic complaints." However, this is a difficult diagnosis to establish without investigating each of them, individually.

The point, of course, is that unless every one of them is listed and evaluated there is no way of knowing which of them is a result of anxiety and which of other underlying medical illness. At the present time, these patients have their problems arranged in priority according to the specialty interest of the doctor they choose to see. If they choose a gynecologist they are evaluated for dyspareunia with headache and backache noted incidentally. An orthopedist focuses, however, on the backache and a neurologist on the headache with the dyspareunia noted incidentally.

By not creating a full data base and problem list, the result for the patient is that he ends up seeing a host of specialists at great cost in order to have his problems evaluated individually. By listing all problems, diagnostic clusters may appear which were not initially obvious.

Such patients present a difficult challenge to the physician. But it is more likely that they will get the care they need when the full data base and problem list are constructed than when their individual problems are treated out of context.

3. The problem-oriented record demands too much data. No one in the busy practice of medicine can spend that much time gathering data and then tracking down every complaint. When the physician listens to a patient history, he makes judgments based on his experience as to which complaints are important and which are trivial.

Ans: Each of these statements deserves a separate answer.

a. The problem-oriented record makes *no* demands about the *size* of the data base, merely that the data base be precisely defined. If the data base is not complete, problem No. 1 should always be "incomplete data base," so that the physician is at least alerted that all information about the patient has not been obtained. As more data is acquired during subsequent visits, the problem list can be expanded appropriately.

b. If the physician's time is limited, he should establish priorities and direct attention to those problems having the greatest potential for moving into the acute phase. The rule should be: When the physician is under pressure, he should do what he does very well; he should select the problem or problems for immediate action, and he should never attempt to deal with all the problems superficially for the mere sake of having dealt with them.

If this approach is followed, the work reflected in each titled progress note can become a precisely defined building block, all effort can be cumulative, and sharply increased efficiency can result.

Ultimately, the argument of "not enough time" is an argument for the hiring of paramedicals to perform such tasks as gathering the data base, relieving the physician to channel his talents into other aspects of clinical care.

Readers who feel that the problem-oriented record is too demanding to be used in medical practice should read *Problem Oriented Practice* by John C. Bjorn, M.D., and Harold D. Cross, M.D.

c. There is no area in medicine which has been less effective than quality control (audit). The physician who feels that his judgment is an adequate substitute for a carefully maintained medical record is setting his own standard and then deciding himself how well he lives up to it. The question is, how does he know how good his judgment is, since no one ever audits his medical records?

There is, of course, at present a quality control of sorts for errors in management of identified problems (errors of commission). But one does not want to be in the position of criticizing one physician for mismanaging a problem which he has at least bothered to find, while another physician is not criticized because he did not find the problem in the first place, or never recorded it (errors of omission).

No physician has ever been able to give total care by himself, without the advice of other colleagues. It is naive to expect that anyone has sufficient experience or memory to decide which problems can be dismissed as unimportant before they are investigated.

4. A specialist certainly does not have the time to create a complete problem list.

Ans: If the specialist is functioning as a consultant he should be presented with a complete problem list by the referring physician; otherwise he will be considering the specialty problem out of context.

If, with a particular patient, he finds himself functioning as a primary-care physician, he should either refer the patient to someone who does have the time to create a complete data base and problem list, or else do it himself as outlined in the answer to the previous question.

5. When computers or paramedical personnel take a patient's history, the non-verbal communication between doctor and patient is lost.

   Ans: a. Because a computer or a paramedical takes the history does not mean that the physician cannot repeat in the presence of the patient those parts of the history that seem to require personal communication.

   b. It is true that non-verbal communication is an important part of patient-physician contact. But it is a mistake to think that all of this communication is beneficial to eliciting a full history. Also communicated to the patient is the fact that the physician may be busy, or not listening closely. Or the patient may feel that the physician does not want to be bothered about this minor problem, when he is being consulted for this other important problem.

   c. When computer-obtained histories have been compared with histories obtained from the same patient by a conscientious physician, the results were quite contrary to the supposed benefits of human contact in history-taking. The number of facts elicited by the physician and not the computer was quite small. But most importantly, the sorts of information that are supposedly best transmitted from one person to another, namely emotional responses, were uncommon in the physician's record but elaborated in detail in the computerized record.

The reason for this is probably that the patient feels no time constraint when entering his own record into the computer. The computer does not become impatient, and no item is too trivial to be recorded.

The computer is not the doctor. As has been written many times, it is a tool, albeit a very powerful one. But when used effectively it can function as an extension of the physician's mind, much as the automobile is clearly an extension of one's muscles.

It may be upsetting to the world's best mind that a mediocre intellect can outperform it when coupled to the right equipment, but that is a reality that many will have to get used to. No one is upset that a 70-year-old arthritic man can ride in a car faster than the best athlete can run. And it is easy to get used to, if you worry more about getting jobs done thoroughly, accurately, and efficiently, and getting good medical care to many people than you do about who it is that does the job.

6. What about emergency situations?

   Ans: It is often thought that a medical record is primarily a record of practice, not the practice itself, and that concern over the record has become a cult for the formulation of charts to the detriment of actually practicing medicine, but this view is correctly challenged in "Better Records: First Step to Better Quality" by Stuart Graves, *Modern Hospital,* April 1971.

   To quote Graves, "In the case of medicine, the word 'record' is misleading; it is not a discrete, separate, precise picture of the reality, medicine. The record is an integral part of that reality which shapes as much as it is shaped. It is a *tool,* the school of thought by which the physician intervenes in the natural history of events. A tool is not a record of reality, it is the handle the practitioner has on reality. . . . Different knowledge of reality produces different behavior practices. Therefore, different medical records create different medical practices. The importance of the medical record is that it determines the very nature of medicine."

If the medical record is an important tool in the practice of medicine, the one time that you certainly don't want to throw away any tools is in an emergency. Some of the most careful records in medicine are found in intensive care units, in emergency rooms (when well run), and at surgery. All that is necessary is to assign someone to keep a record of what is happening. A quickly drawn flowsheet is ideal, on which the parameters being followed (vital signs, drugs administered, etc.) are plotted against time. In this manner it will be abundantly clear what the patient's progress is and what should be done next.

7. Will the problem-oriented record improve the quality of medical care?

   Ans: The problem-oriented record was designed to *assess* the quality of medical care, to organize the recording of medical information so that its quality can be measured. It cannot by itself guarantee quality.

   As stated previously, the medical record is a tool. But it is not the doctor. Giving a chisel and marble to many individuals does not mean that any of them will be Michelangelo, but even Michelangelo cannot scrape away the marble with his fingernails. He needs to use the chisel.

   The current source-oriented record cannot be used as a tool to measure quality, because source orientation destroys the inherent logic of medical decisions.

   The problem-oriented record, by emphasizing precise

statements in entering data and by preserving the logical flow of medical thinking, provides an instrument by which quality can be observed and measured.

Once quality can be measured, the real question is *what will be done about deficiencies?* There are three parts to this feedback loop. First, the problem-oriented record, which allows the assessment of quality. Secondly, a system of audit which detects the deficiencies in quality. And thirdly, corrective action taken by the profession whenever deficiencies are found to exist. There is no point in starting down the path of quality control in medicine unless one is prepared to take the third step of leadership and discipline. Further discussion of this point can be found in "Quality Control and the Medical Record" by Lawrence L. Weed, M.D., Archives of Internal Medicine, Vol. 127, Jan. 1971, and in the paper by Graves previously cited.

8. A computer system, especially when many terminals are needed, is extremely expensive. Can the cost of the system ever be justified? Will it ever be cheap enough so that hospitals can reasonably afford both the initial and operating expenses?

   Ans: This is the question most frequently asked about the computer system. It deserves a detailed answer.

   a. *Relative economy*
      If the question of cost is to have any meaning, the computer system must be compared with the present system. Certainly, if we just compare the cost of a computer terminal for entering medical records with pencil and paper for handwritten records, the comparison is ludicrously one-sided. But this is not a legitimate comparison.

      First, for handwritten records, the cost involves not only making the physical records, but also filing the records in the record room and transporting them, and in addition the managerial superstructure which hires the employees, provides them with working space and equipment, and pays their salaries. It has been estimated that *one-third* of a hospital budget is used for information transfer. These may be considered the *direct costs* of the *present* system.

But there are also *indirect costs* such as the cost of missing patients' problems or inadequately managing them so that they must return for repeat hospitalization and the cost of repeating expensive tests and X rays because the patient was inadequately prepared or the initial plan was poorly conceived (e.g., unnecessary barium enemas, patient on wrong diet for metabolic tests).

b. *Synergism*

The computer makes it possible to reduce these indirect costs, because all aspects of patient care are logically arranged in a computerized record which is available instantaneously to any person involved in the patient's care. It is not possible, for example, to send a patient home after the fracture has healed and ignore the dysuria which is on the problem list, or the still-unreturned thyroid test.

A well-designed computer system, furthermore, is synergistic not only with regard to the medical departments involved in patient care, but also with respect to the business office, the laboratories, and the pharmacy.

When all aspects of patient care are placed in the computer, a true picture of hospital costs can be expected to emerge. For example, consider an automated problem-oriented bill. How much did it cost to provide the care that required hospitalization (fractured hip) and how much did it cost to keep the patient in the hospital to have problems evaluated which could have been handled on an outpatient basis? With the current chaotic system of record-keeping, there is almost no way to arrive at meaningful cost estimates of any aspect of patient care.

c. *Speed of information transfer*
Even if it took very much longer to enter the initial plans for hospital work-up (and it really doesn't), a tremendous saving of both time and money can now ensue, as this information is subsequently manipulated at the speed of light.

Example:
Where radiology departments have been connected to computer displays on the wards, there is no need for the radiologists to spend time on the phone answering questions about the results of the morning's X-ray studies with the ward. Once the films are read, the results are entered into the computer and are instantaneously available on any hospital terminal. There is then no need for the ward physician to waste his time calling the radiologist for results; if it is not on the computer display, then it hasn't been read.

d. *Cost of equipment vs. labor costs*
It follows from the above answer that there may be saving in physician time and the time of other personnel (which is a significant cost) when a computer system is properly used. This cost too must be considered when compared with the cost of equipment.

e. *Audit, quality, and the value of information*
Finally, let us assume for the sake of argument that the computer system is more expensive than current systems (or non-systems). The question really then is, "Is it worth the price?" After all, the reason computerization is being considered in the first place is that the present methods have led to an inadequate health-care system, where both patient and physician satisfaction have been seriously impaired; where the explosion of medical information has put an impossible burden on the physician's memory and

thereby resulted in specialization; and where the current chaotic system of record-keeping has made information transfer a major problem.

Is it worth having logically organized physician's records whose quality may be audited to see that certain standards are being met? Is it worth having a tool which makes the measurement of quality a feasible undertaking? Is it worth having information about costs of hospitalization and outpatient care in a form where they can be compared and meaningful decisions made about them? Is the promise made by hospitals to each patient about quality medical care to have any meaning?

Perhaps the consumer should decide. The consumer makes choices like this every day. Should he buy a Cadillac or a Volkswagen, rent an apartment or buy a house, etc. Similarly, would you rather pay slightly more for quality controlled, total care; or does your present level of care seem satisfactory?

If a decision about computerization is to be made, the following economic considerations should be considered:

i. Is it more expensive than the present system when the full cost of the present system is computed?

ii. Is the cost of the doctor's time being considered?

iii. Are equipment costs being separated into initial costs and maintenance costs; and over how many years should the initial costs be amortized?

iv. Is there a value to information and to quality control?

v. And, perhaps most important, is the computer system based on a philosophy that makes economical, total patient care an achievable reality which can be measured?

9. Can the problem-oriented medical record and computer system substitute for the physician's memory?

Ans: a. *Memory as a pitfall in medical education*

In the past, medical students and physicians have memorized, and been examined on, a large core of medical knowledge. This information was committed to memory in the hope that it would be available at some later date when it would be needed. It was expected that physicians would remember the core information presented in medical school and graduate training and would modify it with the newer information appearing in journals and presented at medical meetings.

But therein lay the trap. No individual's memory was large enough to remember all the facts he might ever need to know. It was found that those facts which were used over and over again could be reliably remembered, but what had been committed to memory and then never used was frequently recalled in an unreliable fashion. It was implicitly recognized that usage determines memory and that performance rather than written examination is the criterion of how well something is remembered. And so physicians, seeking to reduce the amount of information they needed to know, unconsciously resorted to specialization with resultant loss of total patient care.

To reduce further the amount of data to be committed to memory, physicians have relied on patient charts to recall clinical data, libraries for knowledge beyond their experience, and review articles and refresher courses for patching up what has been forgotten.

But despite this obvious acknowledgement of the limitations of memory, memorization and examination have retained a sacred place in medicine. Physicians dislike looking up information in front of patients and applaud feats of memory at CPC's and other conferences.

And nowhere is the myth of memory more revered than in medical schools, where students are taught to rely on their memories rather than exposed to the potential dangers of such a reliance. It contradicts the most basic activities of daily life, for usually when something is important to remember (such as the phone numbers of police and fire departments, or of one's physician), the information is written down rather than memorized.

The point is not that there is no place for memory in the system. With constant usage there is no way to avoid memory. But the system should not be *memory-dependent*. That is, total patient care should not be dependent on the memory or initiative of any individual.

Yet each department in a medical school continues to define a basic core of knowledge which students are expected to memorize, disregarding the connection between usage and memory, and ignoring the fact that they themselves may have forgotten the basic core of knowledge in specialties or sciences other than their own.

b. *Memory and the traditional medical record*
It may well be asked how such a state of affairs could have occurred. How can it be that for fifty years physicians have practiced medicine by relying on memories, and now it is said that this reliance is undesirable?

The answer is that physicians relied on their memories not because it was desirable but because they had no choice. And the reason for this reliance lies in the traditional medical record. Since old habits die hard, both the record and the need for memory have persisted.

As has been stated previously, the medical record is not a record of practice *but the practice itself*. Because the traditional medical record does not clearly link individual problems with the appropriate plans and results, the *logic of the physician's actions is not preserved*. This destruction of the physician's logic in the record obscures the relation between problems and results, and therefore obscures the relation between theory and practice. As a result the tight feedback loop which should exist between basic science and clinical medicine was broken, principles and practice drifted apart, medical students were taught theory in complete isolation from the clinical situations to which the theory applied, and the physician was forced to rely on memorized facts rather than experience.

Once theory and practice became separated, groups of individuals began to specialize in medical theory in isolation from the practice of medicine, and other individuals specialized within the practice of medicine in isolation from the theory. Medical schools became structured into two years of theory and two years of practice, a situation which forced the student to memorize because he could never complete for himself the essential feedback loop on a given patient. The more he memorized, the less well prepared he seemed for clinical medicine, so he was asked to prepare for a longer period of time, until finally the student became caught in an endless web of memorization and preparation.

c. *The problem-oriented record and the computer*

The problem-oriented medical record preserves both data and logic. The physician who uses it asks himself the following questions: "What are the problems? What do I need to know to solve them?"

The data base contains the information necessary to answer the question "What are the problems?" The physician must now address himself to "What do I need to know to solve them or treat them?" In this way the problem-oriented medical record becomes the coupling agent between the patient and sources of information.

Looked at in this way, the physician's memory becomes just one of the available information sources. The medical library has traditionally been the other major source, and now the computer has become a third, and potentially the most powerful, source.

But like memory, the library and the computer are most useful if they provide information organized in such a way as to be applicable to the needs of a given patient. Traditionally the library has not been organized in this way, and once again, physicians found it easier to memorize information than to have to look it up each time they needed it.

But by organizing information in a computer in a problem-oriented fashion and by coupling a physician to an efficiently designed computer terminal, all the information that a physician needs to know to define problems and treat patients can become immediately available to him.

It is now possible to develop a national library of displays which can be logically linked by computer to provide current information on a large variety of problems. The potential significance of such displays is that it turns the library from a static repository of information into a dynamic information source linked directly to the patient's problems.

The patient should not be dependent on the initiative of any individual to ask the right question or use the right information. Rather, the very tools that the physician uses to do his work (e.g., the computer system) should have built into them the parameters of guidance and the currency of information that he needs to do his work well.

10. What are the implications of the problem-oriented record for medical education?

   Ans: Medical education based on the problem-oriented record couples principles and practice in a natural way acceptable to the student. In so doing it protects the student from the misconceptions and inaccurate generalizations of those who teach him.

   Traditional medical education is based on certain premises which actually interfere with the close

coupling of practice and principles that the problem-
oriented record requires. Their negative effect on the
mind of the student is so great that they must be
stated and dealt with in a definitive manner. These
premises and the responses to them are as follows:

Premise 1: The student's memory and store of medical knowledge are the most important qualities to develop.
Response: This was discussed in Question 9.

Premise 2: Principles and precepts should precede practice. Extended preparation is necessary before students be
allowed to do real work.
Response: Discussed in Question 9.

Premise 3: Basic scientists should be allowed to have an overwhelming influence on the first two years of medical
school without any serious attention to a feedback on
their efforts in terms of the student's ultimate performance as either a physician or a researcher.
Response: Any system without a feedback loop runs wild. Basic
science education needs real problems to control it
and bring it to life for the medical student. A graduate
student in the basic sciences has real problems to provide feedback to him, and that is why the basic science
faculty gravitates to him as their real student. The
problem-oriented medical record becomes the vehicle
to couple basic scientists and medical students in a
real and meaningful relationship.

Premise 4: Teachers must set goals for students in terms of
subjects to cover, articles to read, years to spend, etc.
Teachers should give exams and do the audit.
Response: The problem-oriented record is the vehicle whereby
the patient's problems set the goals for both the
student and the teacher. The student formulates the
plans and seeks to solve the problems, and the teacher
audits his efforts.

Premise 5: The theoretical development of medical students requires expensive facilities and personnel devoted solely to education.

Response: The vast funds diverted into separate buildings and faculties to support this erroneous belief have prevented both the full maturation of clinical medicine into a science practiced in accord with basic scientific principles and the development of the manual and computerized problem-oriented records to facilitate this maturation.

Premise 6: There should be a fixed time for medical school and residency training.

Response: Performance should be the constant, and time the variable, between individuals. The problem-oriented record provides the objective means of evaluating performance.

Premise 7: Knowledge for knowledge's sake is a good thing and the mark of a true intellectual.

Response: This belief has provided a pretext for diverting increasing amounts of student and faculty time away from solving patients' problems. But it has been scientifically unsound (no feedback loop) as well as sociologically unacceptable.

SUMMARY

Medical schools have always had as their implied goal the performance of their students as physicians. Yet it is not their performance as physicians which is audited or examined or used as the criterion for licensure.

Rather, it has been assumed that the student's memory (what he knows) would somehow be related to his abilities as a doctor (what he does). This has been due in part to a confusion of the current facts of basic science with the attitudes of basic science, in part to forgetting that the explosion of theoretical knowledge in medicine arose from real problems, and in part to the fact that it is easier to test memory than evaluate performance.

But we can no longer ignore the disparity between our goals and our methods of teaching. If performance is our goal, then performance should be stressed in our teaching. For each task that a student performs, we should ask: Was he *thorough?* Did he get a complete data base? Was he *reliable?* Can we trust his observations and his dedication to the solution of the patient's problems? Was he *efficient?* Did he complete his tasks in a reasonable amount of time? Was his *analytic sense* sound? Did he identify all the problems and plan for each one properly? Note that we are examining performance in terms of behavior and not in terms of a core of knowledge.

What would a curriculum look like that was based on the problem-oriented record?

It would place students in real situations where they searched for real solutions to real problems. It would teach them to trust what they observe rather than repeat what was in the book. It would develop their confidence in *finding* the solutions to problems when they do not already know them, rather than developing their fear of being asked a question they can't answer. It would teach them to couple basic science to the real clinical situation in which the need for the information arises, and would teach them to extract basic questions leading to research from clinical activity.

The false boundary between theory and practice can be removed, and the separation of clinical medicine and basic science *can* come to an end.

REFERENCES

Lawrence L. Weed, "Medical Records, Patient Care, and Medical Education," *Irish Journal of Medical Science,* 6:271–282, 1964.

Lawrence L. Weed, "Medical Records that Guide and Teach," *New England Journal of Medicine,* 278:593–599 and 652–657, 1968.

Lawrence L. Weed, "What Physicians Worry About: How to Organize Care of Multiple-Problem Patients," *Modern Hospital,* 110:90–94, 1968.

INDEX